Facial Skin Resurfacing

Facial Skin Resurfacing

THOMAS J. BAKER, M.D.

Clinical Professor of Surgery (Plastic),
Department of Surgery, University of Miami School of Medicine,
Miami, Florida

JAMES M. STUZIN, M.D.

Assistant Clinical Professor of Surgery (Plastic),
Department of Surgery, University of Miami School of Medicine,
Miami, Florida

TRACY M. BAKER, M.D.

Instructor in Surgery (Plastic),
Department of Surgery, University of Miami School of Medicine,
Miami, Florida

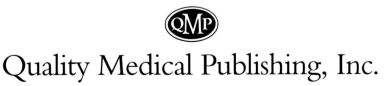

Quality Medical Publishing, Inc.

ST. LOUIS, MISSOURI
1998

Printed in the United States of America.

Illustrations on pp. 5, 6, 8, 55, 56, 60, 87 (top, middle right, bottom right), 89, 94, 101, 105 (middle, right), 109 (bottom), 110 (bottom), 112, 113, 114, 120, 121, 122 (top), 123, 126, 127 (bottom), 129 (top right, bottom), 130 (bottom), 131, 132, 136, 138, 139, 141, 156 (top) from Baker TJ, Gordon HL, Stuzin JM. Surgical Rejuvenation of the Face, 2nd ed. St. Louis: Mosby, 1996.

This book is written for medical professionals, not laymen. Medical knowledge is constantly changing. As new information and equipment become available, indications, technique, results, and complications change. Laser and scanner settings, density, and number of passes are intended as general guidelines only. The thickness of the patient's skin, type of pathology, and color changes with each pass are variables that must be factored into the equation to ensure patient safety and consistent results.

PUBLISHER   Karen Berger

DEVELOPMENTAL EDITOR AND PROJECT MANAGER   Carolita Deter

PRODUCTION   Susan Trail

BOOK DESIGN   Diane M. Beasley and Susan Trail

COVER DESIGN   Diane M. Beasley

COVER ART   David Peace

Quality Medical Publishing, Inc.
11970 Borman Drive, Suite 222
St. Louis, MO 63146

LIBRARY OF CONGRESS CATALOGING-IN-PUBLICATION DATA

Baker, Thomas J.
    Facial skin resurfacing / Thomas J. Baker, James M. Stuzin,
Tracy M. Baker.
        p.   cm.
    Includes bibliographical references and index.
    ISBN 0-942219-77-5
    1. Face—Surgery. 2. Dermabrasion. 3. Chemical peel. 4. Face—
Laser surgery. I. Stuzin, James M. II. Baker, Tracy M. III. Title.
    [DNLM: 1. Skin Diseases—therapy. 2. Skin Aging. 3. Laser
Surgery—methods. 4. Chemexfoliation—methods. 5. Dermabrasion—
methods. 6. Dermatologic Agents—therapeutic use.   WR 650 B168F
1998]
RD523.B347   1998
617.5′20592—dc21
DNLM/DLC
for Library of Congress   97-28725
                                                                        CIP

VT/WW/WW
5   4   3   2   1

Preface

Over the past 30 years we have witnessed dramatic changes in aesthetic surgery. When we first began practice, a face lift involved little more than tightening cheek and neck skin without reelevating facial fat, tightening cervical muscles, or removing facial or cervical fat. Blepharoplasty entailed skin resection or fat removal with little attention paid to brow position, canthal support, or supratarsal crease definition. Facial wrinkling was considered untreatable; wrinkles were thought to be well earned and thus to be endured with dignity.

The present revolution in aesthetic surgery has forever changed our concept of aging. With current techniques, the aging face can be rejuvenated without the traditional sequelae that deterred many would-be candidates from seeking treatment. A youthful appearance can now be recaptured without the stigmata of the "surprised, operated look" so often associated with earlier surgical procedures. We can also offer patients resurfacing procedures that produce smooth, unblemished, youthful-appearing skin for a truly rejuvenated face. Current resurfacing techniques have made a major contribution in this regard, permitting improvement in the quality of the overlying skin cover to enhance the recontoured and anatomically repositioned underlying structures.

Our initial clinical investigations using phenol for treating sun-damaged skin convinced us that chemical peeling could reverse photoaging. Patients were delighted with the results, but our medical colleagues remained skeptical. Concurrently, others were successful in their initial trials using dermabrasion and TCA peeling to reverse the effects of actinic radiation and aging. However, it took almost a decade to convince the medical community of the efficacy of resurfacing. The advantages and limitations of these approaches became obvious with greater clinical experience. It was soon learned that patient selection and precise technique had a major impact on the success of these procedures.

Superficial peeling agents were first introduced in the late 1980s in response to the growing public demand for skin care regimens to improve sun-damaged skin. Today the availability of many different peeling agents and the technologic advances afforded by the pulsed CO_2 laser permit application in a broad spectrum of patients as well as patients with difficult clinical problems once considered intransigent to treatment.

Facial Skin Resurfacing evolved from lessons learned during our 50 years of combined experience with the various modalities for treating facial skin to eradicate the vestiges of aging and sun exposure and ameliorate pathologic skin conditions such as acne scarring and dyschromias. In view of the current media attention and public interest in laser surgery, the latest resurfacing tool, this book is particularly timely and is the first to address all the available options. As we reflect on the advances made in recent decades, it becomes increasingly apparent that no one solution is appropriate for all patients or problems. With so many options now available, physicians must become familiar with superficial, medium-depth, and deep peeling agents and become well versed in using all the current techniques to serve our patients' best interests.

Our writing is based on our personal experience, which has yielded consistent results with a high level of patient satisfaction. These approaches have worked best for us, and we hope that others will benefit from our learning curve. This text should help physicians just starting to treat patients with sun-damaged skin to avoid some of the common pitfalls and develop their own techniques to ensure optimal patient satisfaction.

Starting with the fundamentals that guide the decision-making process, the initial chapters focus on histology and patient consultation and evaluation. A thorough understanding of the histologic changes produced by actinic exposure and the application of the various treatment agents is key to developing a rational treatment plan for photoaging. Before selecting a treatment strategy, consultation and assessment based on skin type and complexion, skin thickness and texture, and degree and level of pathology are requisite. Appropriate clinical decision making depends on these factors as well as an understanding of the patient's needs, lifestyle, and goals. Only then can the best approach be selected for each individual problem area.

The remaining chapters present skin care regimens and specific applications for the three types of resurfacing: chemical, mechanical, and laser. Options, planning decisions, step-by-step procedures, results, and management of complications are discussed in detail. The range of skin care agents and superficial to deep resurfacing techniques is fully explored.

Laser surgery, the newest modality for facial resurfacing, has made it possible to treat patients who were not previously candidates for resurfacing. The final two chapters are devoted to this important topic. As with any new technology, experience is required if consistent results are to be obtained and complications avoided.

• • •

Writing a book is both an exciting and intimidating adventure. One cannot compensate adequately for the time diverted from family and patients. However, the response of those who came to observe our technique and those who attended our courses demonstrates the need to share our clinical experience. As the book progressed, we have been able to put our experience into perspective and gain a greater awareness of how the developmental milestones have influenced the art and science of facial resurfacing. We sincerely hope that the information included in this work will be beneficial to our colleagues and their patients.

Thomas J. Baker
James M. Stuzin
Tracy M. Baker

Contents

Facial Skin Resurfacing

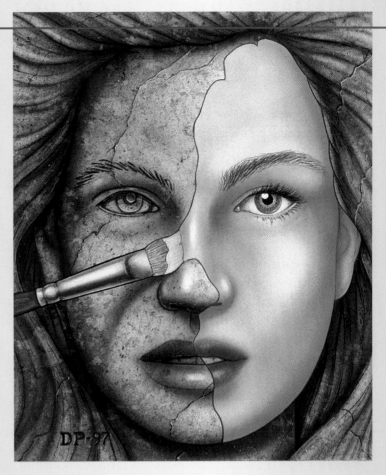

The Evolution of Chemical Peel and Laser Resurfacing

HISTORICAL BACKGROUND

The desire to resurface and restore facial skin is not a new concept. The search for the fountain of youth began long before Ponce de León traveled to the new world. Ancient civilizations worshipped aesthetic beauty and sought remedies to improve appearance and combat aging. Their efforts largely focused on the improvement of surface irregularities, specifically disorders of pigmentation and the treatment of wrinkled skin.

Although there is no recorded evidence of these early efforts, it is likely that prehistoric people used abrasives, oils, and simple herbal remedies derived from plants for treatment of aging skin. The oldest record of cosmetic treatment by physicians is the Ebers Papyrus written around 1560 B.C. that outlined methods for removing wrinkles, dying hair and eyebrows, and correcting squints along with other procedures for body beautification. Early facial resurfacing probably involved certain types of acid treatments. Exfoliation of the skin was accomplished by the direct application of poultices made from mineral and plant substances. Sulfur, mustard, and limestone were also used.

In the early 20th century interest in facial skin resurfacing experienced a revival. As early as 1903 MacKee, a dermatologist, is reported to have used liquefied phenol in the treatment of acne scars. In 1905 Kromayer pioneered the modern use of surgical planing of facial skin and is reported to have used rasps and rotating wheels in the treatment of acne scars, keratoses, and hyperpigmentation. Kromayer, credited as the father of dermabrasion, termed his technique "scarless surgery." Over time this technique evolved from the use of hand-powered instruments to those driven by electric motors incorporating the use of wire brushes and diamond fraises. An astute observer, Kromayer noted that the healing following dermabrasion, as in other forms of facial skin resurfacing, occurred from the epithelium of deep adnexal structures. It was his hypothesis that if resurfacing were not carried below the papillary layer of the dermis, healing would occur without the development of hypertrophic scarring.

The pioneering work of these physicians in the early 1900s was not widely recognized and other early references in the medical literature remain sparse. Greater interest in resurfacing began after World War II. Iverson first noticed favorable results in treating traumatic tattoo injuries by manual abrasion with sandpaper. This led to investigations by McEvitt, who described a similar technique in the treatment of acne scarring. As the cosmetic implications of dermabrasion became appreciated by other dermatologists, interest in facial resurfacing grew in the 1950s. The modern dermabrasion technique was developed by Kurtin in 1953 using a rapidly revolving wire brush following the application of ethyl chloride spray for anesthesia and hardening of the skin. Diamond-impregnated burrs later became popular, allowing the depth of the abrasion to be controlled. As the technical aspects of abrasion improved, the results became predictable and the use of this technique became widespread.

The use of chemical peeling paralleled that of dermabrasion. Because chemical peeling was not applicable to the treatment of battle injuries that occurred in World War II, surgeons took little interest in this modality. Lay clinic operators rather than physicians popularized this technique. During the late 1940s and early 1950s chemical peeling was subject to considerable attention by the news media. These reports proclaimed that the "fountain of youth" had been discovered at last; miraculous results were illustrated in before and after pictures in advertisements by lay clinics. Although facial wrinkles were successfully treated, the medical community remained skeptical. Physicians were quick to condemn these claims as a hoax and were convinced that the case photographs had been retouched.

Medical skepticism, however, did not deter the continuing efforts of some physicians to pursue their investigations of chemical exfoliation. Urkov in 1946 described his method of superficial exfoliation using a mixture of resorcinol and salicylic acid, which became the prototype for light or superficial peels. Another report by Sulzberger in 1961 described treating acne scars with similar chemical agents.

Physicians, however, were forced to acknowledge the remarkable results as they observed growing numbers of patients who had received chemical peels in lay clinics throughout the United States. This stimulated the scientific investigation and evaluation of chemical peeling. Lay operators were loathe to share their "secret" formulas and physicians could gain only scant information about the ingredients.

It is fair to say that plastic surgeons pioneered the investigation of phenol peeling while dermatologists concentrated on the use of trichloroacetic acid in facial resurfacing. Brown, Kaplan, and Brown in 1960 introduced phenol chemical peeling to the plastic surgery literature, although Gillies is reported to have used pure carbolic acid many years previously in a painting and taping technique for the correction of "slight laxity of the lid." However, he did not publish his findings. During this same period Ayres, a dermatologist in California, investigated the effects of trichloroacetic acid on actinically damaged skin as well as the use of dermabrasion in the treatment of epithelial dysplasia.

Following these early reports both plastic surgeons and dermatologists began to use chemical and mechanical resurfacing agents to improve the appearance of sun-damaged skin. The acceptance of these treatment modalities has been gradual and often resisted. It took clinical experience with chemical peeling and dermabrasion and a better understanding of the histology of resurfacing to convince physicians of its merit. As resurfacing agents became more widely used, the indications and limitations of these techniques were delineated and their safety and efficacy improved.

Today a plethora of resurfacing agents have become available. Pharmaceutical investigation of mild acids derived from fruits and vegetables (alpha hydroxy acids and kojic acid) has led to a host of over-the-counter products available for daily skin care and superficial peeling. A greater knowledge of skin biology and the use of retinoic acid in influencing epidermal metabolism have improved the predictability of medium and deep resurfacing agents. With the addition of hydroquinone for influencing melanocytic metabolism, physicians can now apply resurfacing agents to a broad spectrum of patients. The technologic improvements in the CO_2 laser, providing precision in optical penetration and control of thermal injury, offer a new modality that allows deep resurfacing in patients of many skin types. The versatility of these new treatment modalities enables physicians to improve actinically damaged skin in virtually all patients.

MY PERSONAL EXPERIENCE WITH CHEMICAL PEELING

Thomas J. Baker

When I first set up practice in Florida in the 1950s, I encountered many patients who suffered the effects of prolonged sun exposure: fair-skinned individuals with skin cancer, coarse and fine facial wrinkling, and mottled facial pigmentation. We had little to offer these patients except excision of an obvious basal cell carcinoma. Even sunscreens were relatively ineffective at that time, and we knew little about how actinic exposure accelerated the aging process.

My interest in chemical peeling was motivated by my patients who described the miraculous results lay operators in Miami and elsewhere were achieving using secret chemical formulas to remove facial wrinkles and tighten facial skin. The series of articles published by a Chicago newspaper reporter described her experiences with chemical peel and included remarkable before and after photographs. She looked incredibly younger. My medical colleagues smiled, convinced this was yet another attempt to dupe the public. Yet I had seen similar results in patients treated at a local lay clinic and felt that greater scientific investigation was warranted.

Phenol chemical peeling probably was introduced to the United States by the daughter of a French physician, Dr. Laglasse. His daughter, Antoinette, was a lay operator in Los Angeles in the 1930s and 1940s who popularized the procedure but kept her formula secret. One of her trainees, Cora Galanti, taught her technique to Miriam Maschak, who operated the House of Renaissance in Miami from the 1950s to the late 1970s. In all probability Maschak's peeling process was similar to that of Antoinette Laglasse and Cora Galanti, although she never revealed the exact technique and the precise formula used.

As I began observing some of Maschak's patients, I became more and more impressed with the results. I decided to visit the House of Renaissance to talk with Maschak. She was cordial and allowed me to observe patients undergoing treatment, look at before and after photographs, and examine one of her employees who had undergone a chemical peel. The results were miraculous. It seemed to me that this "secret" process achieved the impossible.

Although the lay operators were cordial, they remained protective of their formulas. However, the smell of phenol was pervasive during my visits and became the focal point of my own inquiry.

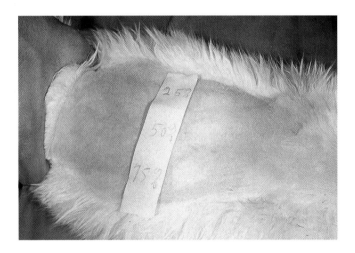

I began the scientific investigation of chemical peeling by examining the effect of phenol applied to rabbit skin in various concentrations. Rapid healing occurred with all concentrations used, although hypopigmentation developed in the test spots treated.

After a series of successful animal studies, I felt confident enough to try this method on human skin. I first applied a 60% phenol solution to an area on my forearm (evidence of this experiment remains to this day).

The second experiment involved a 1 cm area near the hairline of one of the secretaries in our office who readily volunteered. The same formula, a 50% saponified solution, is employed today, the so-called Baker-Gordon phenol peel. The area frosted immediately after this phenol application and reepithelialized in approximately a week. Shortly thereafter she was able to wear makeup over this small erythematous area and eventually it faded and left no sign.

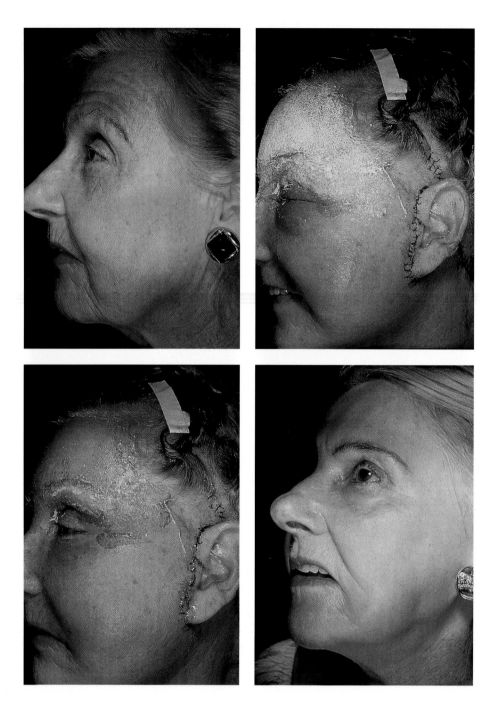

With these two successful applications to human skin, I felt safe in trying this phenol solution on one of our patients, a 69-year-old woman who was undergoing a rhytidectomy. I proceeded to peel the entire forehead after the face lift, rationalizing that if the forehead skin were to slough, a skin graft to the facial unit of the forehead would adequately camouflage it. However, to my delight and amazement the response was extremely good and the patient healed with a smooth, unlined forehead after treatment. Once she had recovered I treated the remainder of her face and the postoperative result was highly satisfactory.

My second experience involved the nursing supervisor of the hospital where we performed most of our surgery. Her results were also excellent and fortified our conviction that chemical peeling was a reproducible method for resurfacing sun-damaged skin.

We then began to use phenol peeling to treat a broad spectrum of dermatologic conditions. By trial and error we found that phenol was primarily useful for coarse and fine facial rhytides and for facial pigmentation problems. As we learned more about the hypopigmentation subsequent to phenol peel, we followed more stringent patient selection guidelines, particularly for regional peeling.

Although the early results with phenol peeling were good, patients with severe actinic damage showed limited improvement. Drawing on the experience of lay operators, we began to use occlusive dressings on a routine basis. A waterproof tape mask became the standard dressing used in the majority of chemical peel procedures performed for 25 years, but today we favor a milder form of occlusion for most patients (a thick layer of Vaseline).

Despite the early results, the plastic surgery community was slow to accept chemical peeling. My first article, published in the *Journal of the Florida Medical Association* in 1961, was entitled "Ablation of Rhytides by Chemical Means." This was followed by the first article on phenol peeling in *Plastic & Reconstructive Surgery* in 1962 entitled "Chemical Face Peeling and Rhytidectomy." My mentor, Dr. Truman Blocker, advised including peeling in combination with rhytidectomy because he believed the manuscript would not be accepted for publication if it focused on chemical peeling alone since this procedure generated widespread skepticism. Other reports in the literature soon followed: Litton (1962) and later Batstone and Millard (1968) added to the growing evidence that chemical peeling was a viable medical treatment. Nonetheless our presentations at plastic surgery symposia were still met with doubt and ridicule.

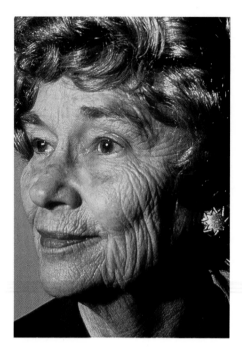 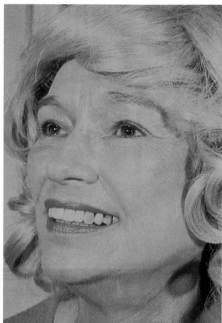

In the face of continued opposition we decided to resort to unorthodox measures. After presenting a paper to the American Society of Plastic and Reconstructive Surgeons in Las Vegas in 1972, we brought out one of our patients who had undergone a face lift, blepharoplasty, and subsequent full-face phenol peel. The participants at this meeting were then invited to come to the podium and examine and question this patient. After seeing the dramatic results of facial resurfacing firsthand, their doubts and skepticism faded. This graphic demonstration was a turning point, and facial resurfacing began to be widely accepted within the medical community.

Since that time there have been many innovations in facial resurfacing that have resulted from knowledge shared between dermatologists and plastic surgeons and the growing public demand for skin rejuvenation. For example, in our practice we once relied on phenol peeling and occasionally dermabrasion but now have expanded to a wide range of agents. Today we routinely use superficial peeling agents, trichloroacetic acid, and laser resurfacing in addition to phenol and dermabrasion. This has allowed us to treat a broader spectrum of patients with more predictable results and often with less morbidity. We have also added an aesthetician to our staff to assist in skin evaluation, formulation of daily skin care regimens, and postoperative camouflaging makeup.

Our approach to skin care has obviously changed with time. In many respects our practice style parallels the approach dermatologists have used for many years in that we now offer superficial and medium-depth peeling in addition to deep resurfacing agents. In a similar fashion, with the availability of the CO_2 laser, many dermatologists now find themselves performing deep resurfacing and treating patients they would have avoided in years past. Essentially skin care and resurfacing have become multidisciplinary, and this sharing of knowledge among the various specialties has produced the dramatic improvement in results we currently see. It is an exciting time to be involved in facial resurfacing. No longer are these techniques the province of a handful of physicians. Now many specialties are involved in treating an ever-growing number of patients. This energy has fueled a momentum and enthusiasm that I believe will carry us forward for many years and ultimately allow us to both intrinsically and clinically transform aged, damaged skin into rejuvenated, youthful-appearing, and architecturally young facial skin.

Concluding Thoughts

Physicians attempting to learn skin care and facial resurfacing today have so many treatment options available that it is difficult for them to master all techniques. Nonetheless, to best serve their patients the physicians must become knowledgeable about the various treatment options available so that the method of resurfacing can be tailored to the needs and desires of the patient. The key to safety and precision in facial resurfacing remains proper patient selection, knowledge of the histologic effects of the various treatment agents, and the proper technical application of the chosen treatment modality. Experience and diligence in pursuing excellence are requisite to mastering resurfacing procedures. In learning these techniques we urge conservatism, especially when deep resurfacing agents are used. All resurfacing procedures can potentially result in hypertrophic scarring. Until the technique is mastered and the physician gains the experience required to adequately judge the depth of penetration required to treat a particular patient's pathology, it is better to err on the side of undertreatment.

Achieving excellent results stems from experience and the critical evaluation of that experience. Pre- and postoperative photographs are essential. Although the artistry and technical mastery of resurfacing techniques are less demanding than those involved in surgical rejuvenation of the face, precise judgment is equally critical. Understanding the modalities available, the depth of pathology to be treated, and maintaining a critical though conservative attitude will allow physicians to progressively and predictably improve results, increasing both patient and physician satisfaction.

REFERENCES

Ayres S. Dermal changes following application of chemical cauterants to aging skin (superficial chemosurgery). Arch Dermatol 82:578, 1960.

Ayres S. Superficial chemosurgery in treating aging skin. Arch Dermatol 85:385, 1962.

Ayres S. Superficial chemosurgery: Its current status and relationship to dermabrasion. Arch Dermatol 89:395, 1964.

Baker TJ. The ablation of rhytides by chemical means: A preliminary report. J Fla Med Assoc 47:451, 1961.

Baker TJ. Chemical face peeling and rhytidectomy. A combined approach for face rejuvenation. Plast Reconstr Surg 29:199, 1962.

Baker TJ, Gordon HL. Chemical face peeling, an adjunct to surgical face lifting. South Med J 56: 412, 1963.

Baker TJ, Gordon HL. Chemical face peeling. In Surgical Rejuvenation of the Face. St. Louis: CV Mosby, 1986, p 37.

Baker TJ, Stuzin JM. Chemical peeling and dermabrasion. In McCarthy JG, ed. Plastic Surgery. Philadelphia: WB Saunders, 1990, p 748.

Baker TJ, Gordon HL, Seckinger DL. A second look at chemical face peeling. Plast Reconstr Surg 37:487, 1966.

Baker TJ, Gordon HL, Stuzin JM. Chemical peeling (phenol and trichloroacetic acid) and dermabrasion. In Surgical Rejuvenation of the Face, 2nd ed. St. Louis: Mosby, 1996, p 45.

Baker TJ, Gordon HL, Mosienko P, Seckinger DL. Long-term histological study of skin after chemical face peeling. Plast Reconstr Surg 53:522, 1974.

Bames HO. Truth and fallacies of face peeling and face lifting. Med J Rec 126:86, 1927.

Batstone JHT, Millard DR Jr. An endorsement of facial chemo-surgery. Br J Plast Surg 21:193, 1968.

Brown AM, Kaplan LM, Brown ME. Phenol-induced histological skin changes: Hazards, techniques, and uses. Br J Plast Surg 13:158, 1960.

Brown AM, Kaplan LM, Brown ME. Cutaneous alterations induced by phenol: A histologic bioassay. Int Surg 34:602, 1960.

Combes FC, Sperber PA, Reisch M. Dermal defects: Treatment by a chemical agent. NY Physicians Am Med 55:36,1960.

Ebbell B (translator). The Papyrus Ebers: The Greatest Egyptian Medical Document. Copenhagen: Levin & Munksgaard, 1937.

Gillies HD, Millard DR. The Principles and Art of Plastic Surgery. Boston: Little, Brown, 1957, p 493.

Litton C. Chemical face lifting. Plast Reconstr Surg 29:371, 1962.

Litton C. Follow-up study of chemosurgery. South Med J 50:1007, 1966.

Litton C, Trinidad G. Complications of chemical face peeling as evaluated by a questionnaire. Plast Reconstr Surg 67:738, 1981.

Litton C, Fournier P, Capinpin A. A survey of chemical peeling of the face. Plast Reconstr Surg 51: 645, 1973.

MacKee GM, Karp FL. The treatment of post-acne scars with phenol. Br J Dermatol 64:456, 1952.

Sperber PA. Chemexfoliation: A new term in cosmetic therapy. J Am Geriatr Soc 11:58, 1963.

Sperber PA. Chemexfoliation for aging skin and acne scarring. Arch Otolaryngol 81:278, 1965.

Sulzberger MB. Dermatology: Diagnosis and Treatment, 2nd ed. Chicago: Year Book, 1961.

Urkov JC. Surface defects of skin treated by controlled exfoliation. Ill Med J 89:75, 1946.

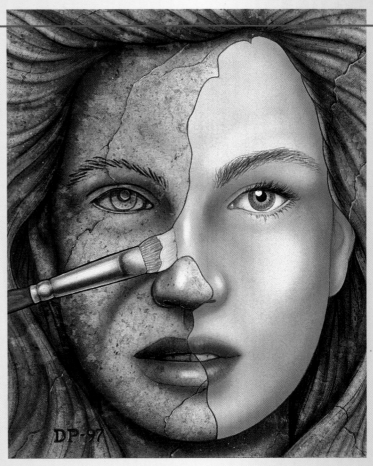

Histologic Effects of Photoaging and Facial Resurfacing

Patients who request skin resurfacing are usually middle-aged women with skin that has undergone actinic damage resulting in degenerative changes in both the dermis and epidermis. The histologic changes of intrinsic aging are similar to those occurring in response to actinic damage. The differences are perhaps more quantitative than qualitative since more accelerated and severe changes are seen in persons who have experienced chronic sun exposure.

In middle-aged patients, photoaging from repeated exposure to ultraviolet light parallels the process of intrinsic aging, the normal aging process that occurs in both exposed and unexposed regions of the body. The visible changes of photoaging are fine and coarse rhytides, surface irregularities, telangiectasias, and pigmentary mottling (the hallmark of melasma secondary to actinic exposure). These changes occur in combination with epidermal dysplasia, which can first be seen as premalignant lesions (actinic keratoses) and can progress to basal cell or squamous cell carcinoma. Histologic changes associated with photoaging include irregularly dispersed melanocytes, solar lentigines, epidermal hyperplasia, and epidermal atrophy associated with loss of vertical polarity in the epidermis. Dermal changes include degeneration of dermal collagen and elastic fibers, a process termed dermoelastosis.

Intrinsically aged skin shows similar changes, including fine wrinkling, dermal atrophy with degeneration of dermal elastic fibers and collagen, and atrophy of subcutaneous facial fat. Thus both intrinsically aged skin and actinically damaged skin show loss of dermal collagen and elastic fibers, but in photoaged skin this process is accelerated and more severe and epidermal dysplasia is more commonly seen.

The histologic changes that occur with aging and actinic exposure are responsible for the clinical manifestations of facial wrinkling, laxity, and mottled pigmentation commonly seen in patients who request skin resurfacing. Mottled pigmentation within the epidermis results from melanin-laden keratinocytes clustering together in the basal layer of melanocytes to form solar lentigines.

Chemical peeling and laser resurfacing can obliterate many of these epithelial lesions and create a new superficial dermis if the proper agent is used and the depth of wounding is adequate. The depth of the histologic changes in actinically damaged skin and the histologic effects of the various peeling agents must be appreciated if skin resurfacing is to be successful.

DEPTH OF PENETRATION OF PEELING AGENTS AND CLINICAL RECOVERY

Numerous chemical agents are currently available for treating actinically damaged skin and are selected based on their depth of penetration. Superficial peeling agents such as Jessner's solution (resorcinol, salicylic acid, and lactic acid), Unna's paste (resorcinol and zinc oxide), salicylic acid, and the alpha hydroxy acids predominantly penetrate the epidermis down to the level of the epidermal-dermal junction. These peeling agents are effective for treating actinic-induced changes in the epidermis, including epidermal dysplasia and pigmentation. Peels at this level produce limited histologic changes, and frequent repeeling is required to produce clinically significant improvement. The advantage of superficial peels is the minimal postpeel morbidity.

Peels that penetrate deep to the dermal-epidermal junction, specifically within the papillary dermis, are commonly termed medium-depth peels. The most commonly used medium-depth agent is 35% trichloroacetic acid. Numerous techniques can be used to increase the penetration of trichloroacetic acid. These include increasing the concentration, applying multiple coats, and using pretreatment agents such as retinoic acid or Jessner's solution. Medium-depth peeling that penetrates the papillary dermis or the upper portion of the reticular dermis not only improves actinically damaged epidermis but also can help reverse damage in the upper dermis. Medium-depth peeling is effective for treating epidermal dysplasia, pigmentary problems confined to both the epidermis and upper dermis, and fine facial wrinkles. The degree of neocollagen formation associated with these peels is minor compared with that afforded by the deep peeling modalities such as phenol, dermabrasion, or laser resurfacing. Medium-depth peeling is associated with a short period of desquamation and reepithelialization within 5 to 7 days. Postpeel erythema usually resolves in less than 2 weeks.

Phenol peeling, dermabrasion, and laser resurfacing represent deep peeling modalities that penetrate into the upper to midreticular dermis and are associated with profound changes following healing. We reserve the use of these treatment agents for patients with severely damaged facial skin. In general deep resurfacing agents are useful for improving epithelial dysplasia resulting from prolonged actinic exposure, blotchy hyperpigmentation associated with melanocytic hypertrophy, and both coarse and fine facial rhytides. Historically, the greatest experience with deep resurfacing for actinically damaged skin has been with phenol peeling. Dermabrasion has been used predominantly for perioral resurfacing and, when used for full-facial resurfacing, has largely been used to treat acne scarring. The advent of the high-energy pulsed CO_2 laser has provided another modality for improving facial wrinkling and actinic damage while minimizing the possibility of posttreatment hypopigmentation.

Because of the significant degree of wounding associated with deep peeling using any modality, there is a greater degree of postpeel morbidity. Desquamation of the epidermis and dermis lead to open oozing wounds that typically last for 7 to 10 days. In general the period of healing and reepithelialization correlates to the depth of the injury. These patients will also experience a prolonged period of posttreatment erythema ranging from 4 to 8 weeks following dermabrasion and up to 4 months following phenol peeling or laser resurfacing.

COMPARISON OF PENETRATION OF SPECIFIC PEELING AGENTS

Patient selection and the ability of the physician to individualize the treatment plan to the specific needs and desires of the patient are key to consistently successful results in facial resurfacing. Some patients prefer the minimal postpeel morbidity accompanying superficial peeling and are willing to undergo the necessary retreatment at regular intervals. For individuals such as these, superficial peels are ideal. In the properly selected patient whose pathologic changes are predominantly confined to the epidermis, these treatment modalities are quite useful.

Other patients whose pathologic changes are localized to the epidermis and the upper portion of the dermis are good candidates for medium-depth peeling. Although the results of medium-depth peeling are not as spectacular as those seen in patients who have deep peels, the improvement can be significant with minor postpeel morbidity.

We reserve deep peeling for patients with significant actinic damage manifest as coarse facial wrinkling or problems of pigmentation confined to the deeper dermis. These agents produce the most dramatic and predictable results but more significant postpeel morbidity; therefore candidates must be highly motivated.

Selecting the most appropriate agent for a patient depends on understanding the histologic response to superficial, medium-depth, and deep wounding agents and the histologic changes that will occur with healing.

Alpha Hydroxy Acids

Alpha hydroxy acids (AHAs) are naturally occurring substances found in many foods. Glycolic acid, which is derived from sugar cane, is the most commonly used agent for superficial peeling. Glycolic acid is highly soluble in water and is a component of many facial creams in concentrations of 10% to 14%. When used as a superficial peeling agent, a concentration of 35% to 75% is used. A greater depth of wounding can be achieved by using greater concentrations of glycolic acid and by increasing the time of exposure.

Epidermal dysplasia subsequent to actinic exposure is associated with hyper-keratinization and excessive corneocyte cohesion. Even low concentrations of glycolic acid will reduce corneocyte adhesion and cause thinning of the stratum corneum. Textural changes in facial skin are noted because of the thinning of the keratin layer of the epidermis after glycolic acid application. Thinning of the stratum corneum also improves the penetration of creams such as Retin-A and hydroquinone, which can be used in conjunction with glycolic acids for treatment of melanocytic hypertrophy resulting in hyperpigmentation.

In addition to improved skin texture, many patients who apply glycolic acid daily will show an improvement in fine wrinkling, especially in the periorbital region. The mechanism of action is unclear, but most likely the low concentrations of glycolic acid do not cause regeneration of dermal collagen. Application of glycolic acids is thought to increase stratum corneum hydration by synthesis of cellular ground substances such as the glycosaminoglycans. Fine epidermal wrinkling will improve with hydration of the epidermis, but these effects are transient and the wrinkles commonly reappear when glycolic acid is discontinued.

By increasing the concentration of the glycolic acid and increasing the length of time the acid remains in contact with facial skin, deeper peeling can be achieved, although rarely will a glycolic acid peel penetrate deep to the dermal-epidermal junction. Concentrations of 70% glycolic acid applied to facial skin for up to 7 minutes usually do not penetrate into the papillary dermis in most patients. If exposure time is increased to provoke epidermolysis, desquamation followed by postpeel erythema may occur. This is rare in our experience. The depth of penetration associated with even 70% glycolic acid solution is such that most of our patients report no change in their daily activities after treatment. Repeating these peels at regular intervals over a period of several months, especially with daily application of lower concentrations of glycolic acid, will produce moderate improvement in skin texture as well as fine facial wrinkling. More impressive is the improved degree of facial pigmentation following daily glycolic use in conjunction with regular application of hydroquinone creams. Use of Retin-A, hydroquinone, and glycolic acid followed by superficial peeling with high concentrations of glycolic acid on a regular basis is perhaps most applicable for treatment of superficial disorders of facial pigmentation.

Trichloroacetic Acid

Trichloroacetic acid (TCA) can be used as a superficial, medium-depth, or deep peeling agent. The depth of penetration can be increased by increasing the concentration of TCA or increasing the number of applications. The chemical effects of a concentration of 10% to 20% TCA correspond to those produced by 70% glycolic acid. At a 20% concentration TCA usually penetrates to the level of the dermal-epidermal junction and is not associated with epidermolysis.

If the patient has undergone proper pretreatment with Retin-A, a low concentration of TCA causes mild desquamation for 5 days after its application. If multiple coats of 20% TCA are applied, the depth of penetration will be deep to the dermal-epidermal junction. If a medium-depth peel is planned, we prefer to use a higher concentration of TCA to produce more rapid and controlled peeling.

Much of the data on peel penetration comes from the classic study by Stegman comparing the histologic depth of penetration of 60% TCA, phenol, and dermabrasion. Stegman noted that in the early phases of healing all three agents showed a significant penetration resulting in crust formation followed by desquamation, wound healing, and erythema. Clinically, he observed that TCA produced more shallow wounding than either phenol or dermabrasion with more rapid healing and less postpeel erythema. He also noted that reepithelialization occurred earlier if wounds were left open rather than occluded with tape.

In comparing the depth of penetration of the three agents, Stegman found that 60% TCA produced necrosis of the epidermis with penetration into the papillary dermis. Baker's phenol solution produced necrosis of both the epidermis and papillary dermis with penetration into the upper one third of the reticular dermis. The depth of penetration of dermabrasion was similar to that of Baker's phenol solution when wounds were left open.

Following wounding with any resurfacing agent, neocollagen formation proceeds in the subepidermal region of the dermis, the so-called Grenz zone. Stegman noted that generally the depth of penetration of the agent corresponded to the degree of neocollagen formation. In other words, Stegman believed that the thickness of Grenz zone fibroplasia was directly proportional to the strength of the wounding agent. In his study comparing TCA, phenol, and dermabrasion, Stegman observed that 60% TCA produced the smallest degree of neocollagen formation, whereas occluded Baker's phenol solution produced the greatest degree of collagen regeneration. He noted that the thickness of the Grenz zone following TCA peeling of unprepared skin was approximately a third of that found after treatment with Baker's phenol solution and approximately two thirds of that seen following dermabrasion. Stegman concluded that the depth of penetration of 60% TCA solution on unprepared skin was less than that seen with either phenol or dermabrasion and therefore was associated with quicker healing and with less resultant neocollagen formation. For this reason, TCA peeling is less predictable in improving coarse facial rhytides.

Obviously methods that increase the depth of penetration of TCA will prolong postpeel healing as well as increase neocollagen formation. In a study comparing the various methods of increasing TCA penetration, Brody compared pretreatment with Jessner's solution prior to application of 35% TCA with pretreatment using frozen CO_2 slush. The initial wounding was deeper with frozen CO_2 slush since this agent produces complete epidermal necrosis that allows greater TCA penetration. Histologically, greater TCA penetration produced a moderate degree of neocollagen formation in the upper dermis. In contrast, pretreatment with Jessner's solution followed by a single application of TCA failed to stimulate any detectable neocollagen formation within the upper dermis, as shown by biopsies 90 days following treatment. Brody also demonstrated that pretreatment with frozen CO_2 slush followed by three applications of 35% TCA was associated with even greater penetration as compared with a single TCA application, resulting in augmented dermal collagen formation.

Clinically, TCA penetration of the papillary or upper reticular dermis (medium-depth peeling) is associated with improvement of epidermal actinic degeneration, facial hyperpigmentation, and fine facial wrinkling. Both clinical and histologic studies indicate that neocollagen formation after TCA peeling (especially to a medium depth) is more limited than with either phenol peeling, dermabrasion, or laser resurfacing. The improvement of coarse facial wrinkling is less predictable with this peeling agent. Although most investigators have focused on depth of penetration as the predominant criteria for neocollagen formation following wounding, it has been our experience that TCA peels that penetrate the reticular dermis do not produce the same degree of neocollagen formation obtained with other deep resurfacing agents. The healing response after TCA peeling differs from that observed after phenol peeling. TCA has a more limited effect on melanocytic function as compared with phenol, and its effect on fibroblastic proliferation also appears to be less. Multiple histologic studies confirm that neocollagen formation following wounding with TCA is limited in comparison to phenol or dermabrasion and most likely depth of penetration is only one factor. This may explain the different results obtained with these various resurfacing agents.

Phenol

In our opinion the most predictable results, both histologic and clinical, can be obtained with phenol peeling. A single application of phenol solution (Baker's formula) to unprepared facial skin leads to a predictable degree of dermal penetration followed by a predictable degree of neocollagen formation. To appreciate the histologic effect of phenol in the treatment of actinically damaged skin, the histologic damage that occurs with prolonged actinic exposure must be understood.

Histology of Sun-Damaged and Aging Skin

Epidermis. The epidermis in sun-damaged skin tends to be atrophic and flat. The cells are small and exhibit cellular disarray associated with actinic atypia and dysplasia. Typically there is a loss of vertical polarity signifying a reduction in the normal maturation between the basement membrane and the stratum corneum. The basement membrane usually is thickened, ragged, and blurred.

The melanocytes along the basal layer commonly are more numerous and unevenly distributed. The number of melanin granules within keratinocytes is variable. Some epidermal cells appear to be engorged with dense pigmentation, whereas others are virtually empty. This uneven distribution of melanin explains the blotchiness of photodamaged skin.

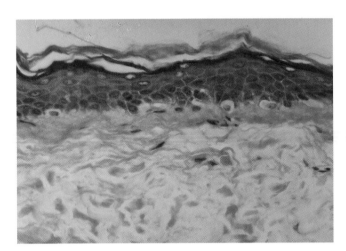 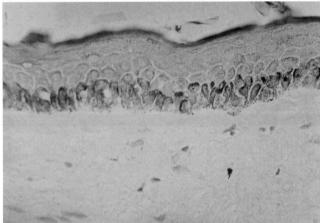

The photomicrograph on the left shows the typical appearance of actinically damaged epidermis. The keratinocytes are variable in size, shape, and staining characteristics, indicating atypia. The granular layer is thin and inconspicuous. The epidermis is atrophic, flat, and exhibits marked dysplasia because of failure to differentiate in an orderly fashion and hence polarity is absent. The histologic specimen on the right demonstrates the typical atrophic appearance of actinically damaged epidermis associated with dense clumping of melanin granules distributed irregularly along the basal layer of the epidermis. Such uneven disposition of melanin accounts for the mottled, blotchy appearance of photoaged skin.

Dermis. Elastosis is the hallmark of sun-damaged skin. It consists of thickened, coiled, tangled, dense masses of altered collagen and elastic fibers. Routine hematoxylin–eosin staining of actinic skin reveals basophilic degeneration of collagen and elastic fibers. Mowry staining shows an increase in ground substance in the form of acid mucopolysaccharides present within the dermis. In general collagenolysis is related to the degree of elastosis and the increase in glycosaminoglycans.

Typically, actinically damaged skin will have a normal-appearing band of collagen just deep to the basement membrane of the epidermis. This region, termed the Grenz zone, represents the area where new collagen is formed by hyperplastic fibroblasts in an attempt to repair the chronic injury from actinic exposure. This region of the dermis immediately below the basal layer of the epidermis is largely responsible for the regenerative changes seen after chemical peeling.

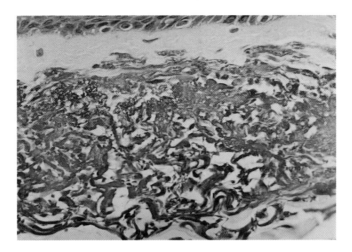

This photomicrograph shows the typical appearance of severely photoaged skin. The entire dermis is occupied by abnormal elastotic tissue representing end-stage deterioration of the elastic fiber and collagen network. Note the small band of normal-appearing subepidermal collagen that is attempting to repair the chronic damage caused by ultraviolet light. This thin band just deep to the basement membrane of the epidermis is the Grenz zone and is a hallmark of actinically damaged dermis.

Histologic Response to Phenol Peeling

The application of phenol produces a controlled chemical injury to the level of the upper reticular dermis, which removes both the damaged epidermis and elastotic upper dermis. On healing the skin rejuvenates. As with other partial-thickness injuries, healing following deep resurfacing proceeds from the epithelial appendages.

Epidermis. The regenerated epidermis exhibits a normal morphology after phenol peeling. Epidermal atrophy and dysplasia are eliminated, and the reconstituted epidermis appears plump as the vertical polarity between the basement membrane and the stratum corneum is restored.

Invariably phenol peeling produces hypopigmentation. Although many investigators thought that phenol had a cytotoxic effect on epidermal melanocytes, histologic studies do not support this. Biopsies of phenol-peeled skin reveal that epidermal melanocytes are still present after resurfacing but are incapable of synthesizing normal amounts of melanin. Close inspection reveals that these melanocytes contain fine pigment granules that are evenly dispersed and show no tendency to clump and form pigmented areas or solar lentigines. Microscopic actinic keratoses are rarely observed following phenol resurfacing.

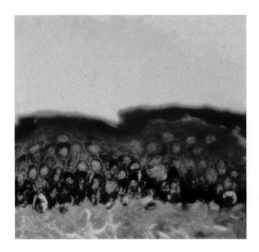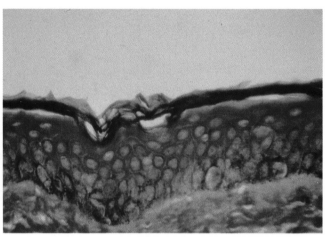

On the left is a photomicrograph of untreated photodamaged epidermis. Note the atrophic appearance of the epidermis with loss of vertical polarity. Also note the clumping of pigment along the basement layer of the epidermis. This histologic appearance corresponds to the clinical manifestation of solar lentigines commonly seen in sun-damaged skin. On the right is a photomicrograph of treated epidermis. The epidermis exhibits normal architecture and correction of atypia following phenol peeling. No clumping of pigment along the basement membrane is seen, as is typical after phenol peeling. The histologic effect of phenol on melanocyte distribution and function is the underlying cause of hypopigmentation following phenol peeling.

Dermis. Biopsies taken 48 hours after phenol peeling demonstrate keratocoagulation necrosis extending into the upper reticular dermis. Epidermal regeneration begins at 48 hours and is usually complete within 7 to 10 days. Dermal regeneration is delayed, and biopsies 2 weeks following phenol peel show incomplete regeneration of the dermis. At 3 months the upper elastotic dermal collagen has been replaced and the architectural arrangement exhibits an organized wavy appearance of parallel collagen bundles characteristic of youthful skin.

Mallory staining following phenol peeling reveals a significant decrease in glycosaminoglycans within the newly reconstituted dermis in conjunction with a significant increase in both collagen and elastic fibers. These newly formed collagen and elastic fibers in association with a diminution in dermal ground substance explain the transition from wrinkled, slack skin to smoother, fuller, and more resilient skin following phenol peeling. In other words, the clinical effects of phenol peeling reflect the remarkable histologic changes seen within the dermis.

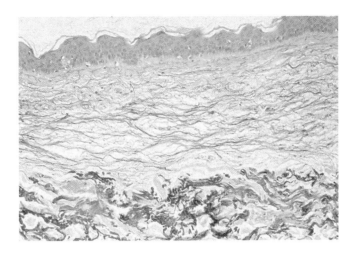

This photomicrograph demonstrates the degree of neocollagen formation typically seen after phenol peeling. Even without pretreatment of facial skin, a single application of phenol solution leads to a predictable degree of penetration of the upper reticular dermis followed by a predictable degree of neocollagen formation. Note the untreated elastotic dermis present at the base of this photomicrograph, which is beyond the limit of solution penetration.

Although the histologic changes are apparent within a few months following healing, distinct differences can be seen in treated skin up to 20 years following chemical peeling. Clinically, few treatment modalities offer long-term effects provided by phenol peeling. Rarely do facial rhytides recur in patients who have undergone phenol peeling. Biopsies of these patients taken several years after phenol resurfacing demonstrate persistence of neocollagen formation despite continued intrinsic aging.

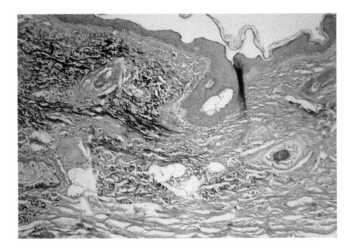

A biopsy specimen several years after a phenol peel shows the line of demarcation between treated and untreated skin. Along the untreated specimen (left side) note the dermal elastosis typical of sun-damaged skin. In the treated portion (right side) neocollagen formation following phenol peeling is apparent.

Dermabrasion

Dermabrasion is a process in which the epidermis and the upper portion of the dermis are mechanically abraded to a desired depth. The advantage of dermabrasion is that the depth of wounding can be precisely controlled to treat the individual patient's dermal pathology. Stegman showed that dermabrasion produced wounds that were comparable to those produced by Baker's phenol solution, although the resulting edema did not extend as deeply into the dermis as with phenol. Stegman found that the epidermis was entirely obliterated in this process and that the wounding occurred throughout the entire papillary dermis and into the upper reticular dermis. With phenol the rete ridges in the papillary dermis appeared to be fairly normal, both in number and appearance, after healing. However, dermabrasion results in a decrease in number of and flattening of the rete ridges; the epidermis also appears flattened.

The amount of collagen formed within the Grenz layer following mechanical wounding appears to be similar to that following use of Baker's phenol solution. Melanocytic function is affected to a lesser degree by mechanical abrasion, and for this reason, pigmentation changes after dermabrasion are less of a problem than with phenol. The predictable degree of neocollagen formation following dermabrasion makes it useful for treating actinically damaged facial skin, specifically for improving both coarse and fine facial wrinkling.

Laser Resurfacing

The histologic effects of laser resurfacing are microscopically similar to phenol peeling in the treatment of sun-damaged skin. Unlike phenol peeling in which a single application will produce a predictable degree of dermal penetration, laser resurfacing is dose dependent. Increasing the pulse energy as well as increasing the number of passes produces a greater degree of dermal penetration. When laser resurfacing is carried into the upper reticular dermis, the dermal changes following healing parallel those of phenol. The abnormal elastotic tissue is eliminated and new collagen in the upper dermis is formed. Shortly after wounding, granulation tissue is formed in the usual sequence as macrophages and fibroblasts increase in number and angiogenesis occurs. These inflammatory changes resolve by 6 months after resurfacing, at which time the dermal matrix of new collagen becomes stabilized.

The epidermal changes following laser resurfacing parallel those seen with phenol peeling. Biopsies of resurfaced facial skin reveal a reversal of epidermal atrophy, atypia, and a restoration of vertical polarity. The tendency toward clumping of pigment in the basement membrane of the epidermis typically seen in sun-damaged skin is ameliorated following laser treatment.

The major histologic difference between phenol and laser resurfacing is the pigmentary changes occurring within the epidermis. Phenol peeling does not destroy epidermal melanocytes; however, melanin can no longer be synthesized. This results in permanent hypopigmentation. Laser resurfacing exhibits less long-term effect on melanocytes. Although biopsies demonstrate an absence of clumping of pigment in the basal layer following laser treatment, melanocyte function appears intact. The histologic effect on epidermal melanocytes permits regional laser resurfacing with a diminished risk of an obvious line of demarcation between treated and untreated skin. This makes laser resurfacing applicable to a broader spectrum of patients than phenol peeling.

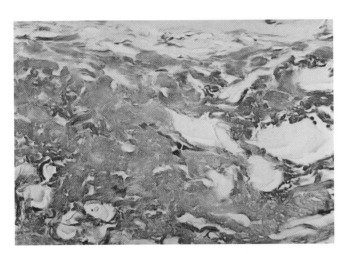 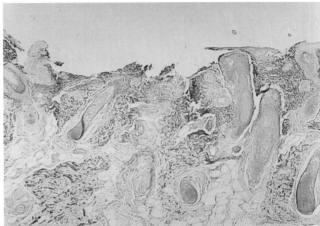

The penetration of laser resurfacing is dose dependent. Increasing pulse energy and increasing the number of passes applied to the skin will increase dermal penetration. The photomicrograph on the left illustrates the immediate effect of two passes using 300 mJ of pulse energy (Coherent UltraPulse CO_2 laser with a 3 mm handpiece and 10% spot size overlap). The epidermis and the underlying Grenz zone have been completely destroyed. The elastotic tissue in the upper dermis shows the coagulative effect of thermal injury. The photomicrograph on the right illustrates the immediate effect of four passes using 500 mJ of pulse energy. The laser energy has penetrated the mid to deep reticular dermis. Penetration to this depth represents the histologic limit of dermal healing without hypertrophic scarring.

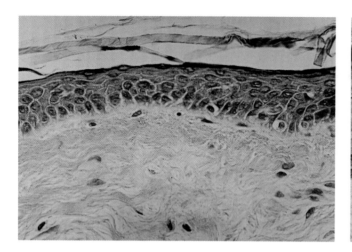 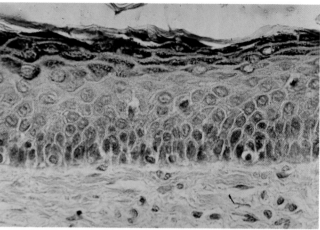

The histologic specimen on the left demonstrates the typical appearance of actinically damaged epidermis. The epidermis is atrophic, flat, and exhibits marked dysplasia from failure to differentiate in an orderly fashion, hence polarity is absent. As seen on the right, the epidermis is thickened and has a prominent granular layer 5 months after laser treatment. Differentiation is complete with elimination of actinic atypia, and the basement layer and the stratum corneum show normal polarity. The keratinocytes are hypertrophic, reflecting the increased proliferative activity and rapid turnover. Clinically, the patient's skin is youthful and smooth.

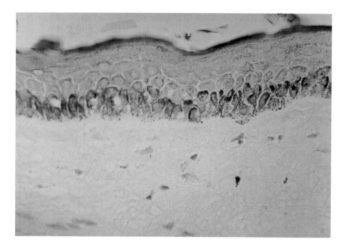 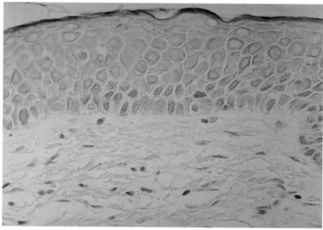

In the photomicrograph on the left the untreated epidermis appears atrophic with dense clumps of melanin granules distributed irregularly along the basal layer of the epidermis. This uneven disposition of melanin accounts for the mottled, blotchy appearance of photoaged skin. In the photomicrograph on the right the polarity is restored and the epidermis appears normal. Melanin granules are sparse and evenly distributed. The elimination of melanocytic hypertrophy after laser resurfacing results in the clinical improvement of blotchy hyperpigmentation commonly seen in photoaged skin.

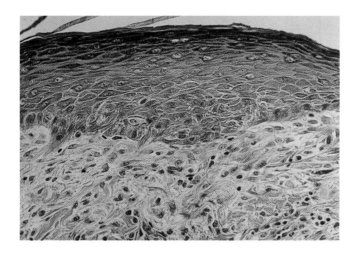

Fifteen days after laser treatment the epidermis has regenerated and the keratinocytes are large and interspersed with large spaces. The dermis is infiltrated with fibroblasts, histiocytes, and lymphocytes. The fibroblastic proliferation noted early after wounding is responsible for the later stable neocollagen formation in the upper dermis, which accounts for the clinical results following laser treatment.

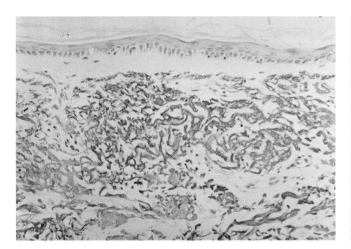 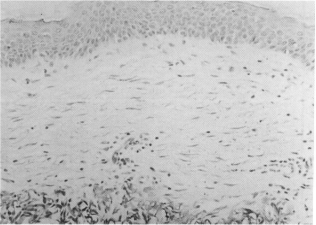

The untreated histologic specimen on the left shows severely photoaged skin. Except for the subepidermal Grenz zone, the entire dermis contains abnormal elastotic tissue representing end-stage deterioration. The photomicrograph on the right shows the histologic changes 3 months after laser treatment. The normal epidermis reveals an absence of epidermal dysplasia and a return of normal polarity. The elastotic mass of the upper to middermis has been completely replaced by normal dermal matrix, signifying regeneration of collagen. Remnants of the old elastotic tissue can be seen in the lowermost portion of this photomicrograph. The new dermis is highly cellular, exhibiting many hypertrophic fibroblasts, along with many new small blood vessels.

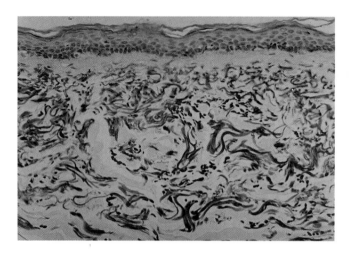 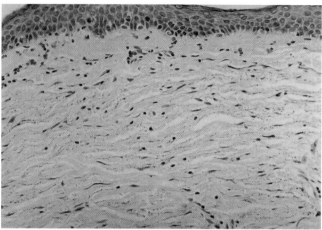

The untreated specimen on the left demonstrates the typical appearance of photoaged skin. Marked elastosis is evident in the deeper dermis and a thin Grenz zone of normal collagen appears beneath the atrophic epidermis. Six months after laser resurfacing the elastotic tissue has been completely replaced by new bundles of normal collagen, as seen on the right. Fibroblasts are numerous. Although not visible here, higher power magnification shows new elastic fibers interspersed among the collagen bundles. The histologic results represent essentially normal epidermis and dermis.

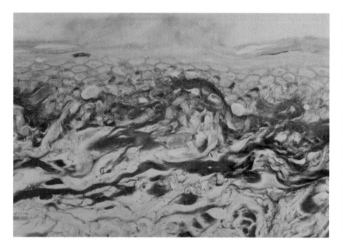 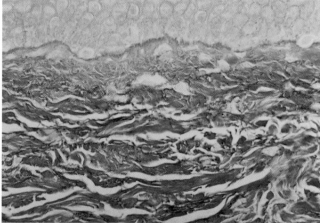

The specimen on the left shows the typical appearance of photoaged skin following Hale staining, which tints collagen red and glycosaminoglycans blue. Note the paucity of collagen in the deeper dermis. The intervening spaces are filled with glycosaminoglycans. The greater amount of ground substance dispersed among the remnants of collagen is typical of advanced photodamage. The specimen on the right taken 6 months following laser resurfacing shows a wide band of new collagen in the upper dermis as well as diminished glycosaminoglycans, accounting for the skin's firmness and clinical improvement of coarse rhytides.

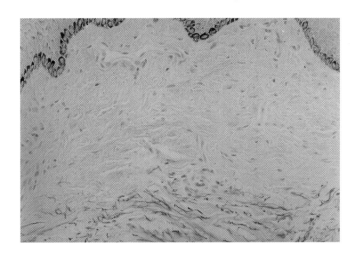

This histologic specimen was taken from a postauricular test site on a black patient 3 months after laser resurfacing. Note the striking degree of neocollagen formation in the upper dermis. The epidermis exhibits the even distribution of epidermal melanocytes along the basement membrane, which retain the ability to synthesize melanin. This is the histologic appearance of youthful black skin.

CONCLUDING THOUGHTS

The histologic effects produced by the various skin resurfacing agents must be thoroughly understood if the physician is to obtain consistent results and ensure overall patient satisfaction. In general the greater the depth of wounding, the greater the degree of neocollagen formation and the greater improvement in the appearance of facial wrinkles. With deeper wounding, however, it will take longer for reepithelialization to occur and erythema will be prolonged. Although depth of penetration is correlated with neocollagen formation, not all peeling agents produce the same degree of neocollagen formation for comparable levels of dermal penetration. Deep resurfacing is often associated with bleaching of facial pigmentation and textural changes of the skin, and this must be factored in when individualizing the treatment plan to the specific needs and desires of the patient, especially when regional treatment modalities are used.

Figures on pp. 18 (right), 23 to 27 from Stuzin JM, Baker TJ, Baker TM, Kligman AM. Histologic effects of the high-energy pulsed CO_2 laser on photoaged skin. Plast Reconstr Surg 99:2036, 1997.

REFERENCES

Ayres S. Dermal changes following application of chemical cauterants to aging skin (superficial chemosurgery). Arch Dermatol 82:578, 1960.

Baker TJ, Gordon HL. Chemical face peeling and dermabrasion. Surg Clin North Am 51:387, 1971.

Baker TJ, Stuzin JM. Chemical peeling and dermabrasion. In McCarthy JG, ed. Plastic Surgery. Philadelphia: WB Saunders, 1990, p 748.

Baker TJ, Gordon HL, Seckinger DL. A second look at chemical face peeling. Plast Reconstr Surg 37:487, 1966.

Baker TJ, Gordon HL, Stuzin JM. Chemical peeling (phenol and trichloroacetic acid) and dermabrasion. In Surgical Rejuvenation of the Face, 2nd ed. St. Louis: Mosby, 1996, p 45.

Baker TJ, Gordon HL, Mosienko P, Seckinger DL. Long-term histological study of skin after chemical face peeling. Plast Reconstr Surg 53:522, 1974.

Brody HJ. Chemical Peeling. St. Louis: Mosby–Year Book, 1992.

Campbell RM. Surgical and chemical planing of the skin. In Converse JM, ed. Reconstructive Plastic Surgery, 2nd ed. Philadelphia: WB Saunders, 1977, p 442.

Cotton J, Hood AF, Gonin R, Deeson WH, Hanke CW. Histologic evaluation of preauricular and postauricular human skin after high energy short pulsed carbon dioxide laser. Arch Dermatol 132:425, 1996.

Fitzpatrick RE, Tope WD, Goldman MP, Satur NM. Pulsed carbon laser, trichloroacetic acid, Baker and Gordon phenol, and dermabrasion: A comparative clinical and histologic study of cutaneous resurfacing in a porcine mode. Arch Dermatol 132:469, 1996.

Kligman AM, Baker TJ, Gordon HL. Long-term histologic follow-up of phenol face peels. Plast Reconstr Surg 75:652, 1985.

Litton C. Chemical face lifting. Plast Reconstr Surg 29:371, 1962.

Montagna W, Carlisle K. Structural changes in aging human skin. J Invest Dermatol 73:47, 1979.

Resnik SS. Chemical peeling with trichloroacetic acid. J Dermatol Surg Oncol 10:549, 1984.

Rudolph R, Woodward M. Ultrastructure of elastosis in facial rhytidectomy skin. Plast Reconstr Surg 67:295, 1981.

Spira M, Dahl C, Freeman R, Gerow FJ, Hardy B. Chemosurgery—A histological study. Plast Reconstr Surg 45:247, 1970.

Stagnone JJ. Chemical peeling and chemabrasion. In Epstein E, ed. Philadelphia: WB Saunders, 1987, p 412.

Stegman SJ. A study of dermabrasion and chemical peels in an animal model. J Dermatol Surg Oncol 6:490, 1980.

Stegman SJ. A comparative histologic study of the effects of three peeling agents and dermabrasion on normal and sun-damaged skin. Aesthetic Plast Surg 6:123, 1982.

Stuzin JM, Baker TJ, Gordon HL. Treatment of photoaging: Facial chemical peeling (phenol and trichloroacetic acid) and dermabrasion. Clin Plast Surg 20:9, 1993.

Stuzin JM, Baker TJ, Baker TM, Kligman AM. Histologic effects of the high-energy pulsed CO_2 laser on photoaged skin. Plast Reconstr Surg 99:2036, 1997.

Wolfort FG, Dalton WE, Hoopes JE. Chemical peel with trichloroacetic acid. Br J Plast Surg 25:333, 1972.

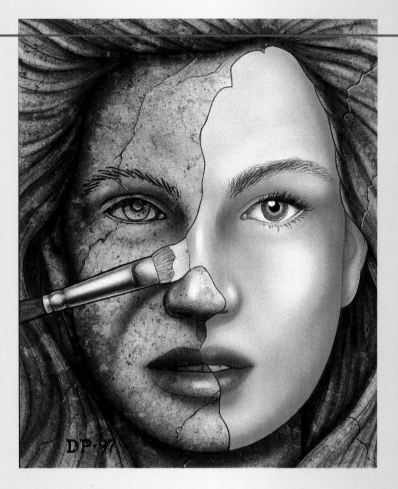

Patient Consultation
and Evaluation

The combined efforts of dermatologists and plastic surgeons have led to innovative approaches to the treatment of patients with environmentally damaged skin and broadened the therapeutic options. The advantages, disadvantages, and indications for these various options must be carefully weighed by both physician and patient so that a rational treatment plan can be developed. As in all aesthetic facial procedures, proper patient evaluation and individualization of treatment are crucial components for a successful outcome. The ability to diagnose the problem and devise a creative aesthetic solution leads to consistently rewarding results. Incorporating the patient's desires and expectations into the surgical treatment plan is key to patient compliance and ultimate satisfaction.

GENERAL INDICATIONS

Chemical peeling and laser resurfacing have well-defined indications. These therapies are not appropriate for all patients or all problems. Careful patient selection is a critical factor. In general resurfacing procedures are particularly effective in treating two clinical conditions: facial wrinkles and blotchy skin pigmentation caused by pregnancy, birth control pills, and chronic sun exposure. As an added benefit, resurfacing procedures regenerate the dysplastic epithelium in patients with sun-damaged skin and actinic keratoses. Deep facial resurfacing is effective for treating the occasional patient who has multiple actinic keratoses and is prone to neoplastic degeneration of facial skin.

Although prior cosmetic surgery is neither a relative contraindication nor indication for chemical peeling or laser resurfacing, it does influence treatment decision making. Interestingly, patients who have undergone prior facial cosmetic procedures are usually more compliant in following a skin care program. These patients recognize that perioperative morbidity may be prolonged and better adapt to the inconveniences associated with medium-depth or deep resurfacing procedures.

Specific problems that must be considered in patients who have undergone previous cosmetic surgery include lower eyelid appearance following blepharoplasty, residual rhytides after a previous resurfacing procedure, and the unresolved signs of actinic damage after a face-lift procedure.

If a patient has developed lower lid retraction after lower lid blepharoplasty, a deep peel of the lower lids must be performed judiciously. These patients are best treated with medium-depth peels or a deep resurfacing procedure performed in conjunction with surgical repair of the lax lower lid. If a patient has undergone chemical peeling or dermabrasion in conjunction with cosmetic surgery, medium-depth or deep peels can still be performed with good results provided skin thickness and texture will permit successful wound healing. In patients with residual upper and lower lip rhytides after a perioral phenol peel, we prefer to use dermabrasion or laser resurfacing as secondary procedures since the depth of the injury can be better controlled. Chemical or CO_2 laser resurfacing generally produce limited results in patients with hypertrophic and burn scars, port-wine stains, and telangiectasias and are not indicated for these problems. Similarly, all but the most superficial acne scars are intransigent to treatment with chemical peeling agents. Dermabrasion or laser resurfacing is a more effective treatment modality for this clinical condition.

CONSULTATION

Numerous factors influence the ultimate success of any facial resurfacing and skin care program, and these must be explored in depth during the initial doctor-patient consultation. Foremost among these are patient expectations and treatment goals. Most patients who seek treatment for facial aging mistakenly assume that some type of face lift will produce the desired improvement regardless of the nature of the problem. Frequently they believe that a face lift will eradicate all facial wrinkles. To them, wrinkles are synonymous with sagging facial skin and descended facial fat and they commonly do not differentiate between the gravitational changes of aging and the effects of photoaging. It is our observation that disorders of photoaged skin are not responsive to surgical therapy. Pigmentary changes, multiple fine and coarse facial rhytides, and acne scarring are perhaps better treated using chemical, mechanical, or photoelectric techniques that address the pathologic photodamage localized to the epidermis and dermis.

The relative benefits of facial resurfacing as opposed to rhytidectomy must be fully explored before a treatment plan is selected. We devote considerable time to defining the differences in available treatment options and the results that can be expected. We tell patients that a face lift improves the visual effects of gravitational and intrinsic aging, whereas resurfacing procedures improve fine lines, creases, and the pigmentary changes in facial skin. Analogous to having a tailor alter a garment, the garment may fit perfectly but still may be marred by wrinkles that require steaming. This steaming process corresponds to the response produced by a resurfacing treatment that smooths fine facial lines. If the patient's goal is to eradicate facial wrinkles and fine lines, this can be accomplished with resurfacing procedures without the need for surgical intervention.

Once the decision is made, we carefully outline the various treatment options available (chemical, mechanical, and photoelectric) ranging from superficial to deep penetration and their relative indications. We also explain the specific steps involved in each modality as well as the required skin treatment regimens and the expected morbidity and recovery (see Chapters 5, 6, 7, and 9 for more specific information). The more informed the patient, the smoother the course of treatment. Although patient education pamphlets, videotapes, and CD-ROMs are useful adjuncts, they are no substitute for verbal communication between the physician and patient with ample opportunity for asking questions and expressing concerns. It also allows the physician to assess nonverbal clues concerning patient expectations, motivation, and willingness to undergo the potential morbidity associated with deeper resurfacing procedures.

In addition to explaining the various skin resurfacing approaches and addressing questions, the surgeon should elicit specific information about the patient's lifestyle such as recreational or occupational activities involving prolonged sun exposure. Since outcome of treatment is directly related to patient compliance, the patient must be willing and able to make lifestyle changes to comply with the requirements of a skin care program, including regular application of Retin-A, hydroquinone, or other prescribed creams; judicious application of sunscreens; and avoidance of sun exposure.

ASSESSMENT

Patient assessment focuses on skin type and complexion, skin texture and thickness, the degree of photoaging and severity of facial rhytides, and age-related gravitational changes. Armed with this information the physician can formulate a systematic treatment plan. Although some pathologic conditions respond better to more aggressive treatment, the lifestyle of the patient may preclude such therapy. The morbidity associated with the procedure must be weighed against the needs and desires of the patient. Only with a thorough understanding of the treatment possibilities and the patient's goals can a satisfactory solution be devised.

SKIN TYPE AND COMPLEXION

By correlating the specific skin type with the patient's complexion (degree of pigmentation) and eye and hair color the physician can more accurately determine which type and concentration of agent will produce the best treatment outcome. We have found the Fitzpatrick classification to be a useful guide for evaluating skin types and response to sun exposure. This classification system ranks the skin's tendency to tan or burn following actinic exposure. In general patients who readily burn but do not tan (skin type I) following sun exposure have a lower incidence of postoperative hyperpigmentation following any resurfacing procedure. Patients who easily tan in response to ultraviolet rays can experience hyperpigmentation subsequent to the dermal injury associated with resurfacing. Conversely, patients with type I skin are more prone to posttreatment hypopigmentation following any form of resurfacing. We stress the need to obtain an accurate history of how patients respond to sun exposure when selecting the treatment options and the pretreatment care required for individual patients.

The patient's complexion or degree of facial pigmentation is influenced by genetic factors and determines the ability of the skin to withstand environmental injury. Patients with Fitzpatrick types I and II skin have a low incidence of

Skin Type, Color, and Reactions to First Summer Exposure

SKIN TYPE I

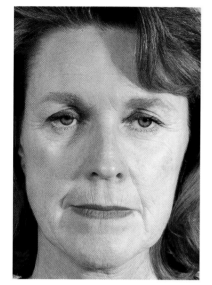

Color: White
Reaction: Always burns, never tans

SKIN TYPE II

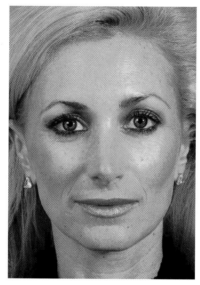

Color: White
Reaction: Usually burns, tans with difficulty

SKIN TYPE III

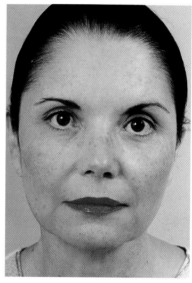

Color: White
Reaction: Sometimes exhibits mild burn, average tan

SKIN TYPE IV

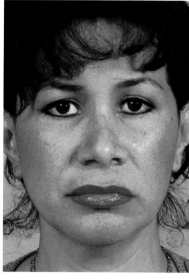

Color: Moderate brown
Reaction: Rarely burns, tans with ease

SKIN TYPE V

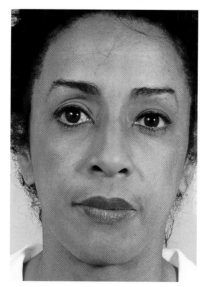

Color: Dark brown*
Reaction: Very rarely burns, tans very easily

SKIN TYPE VI

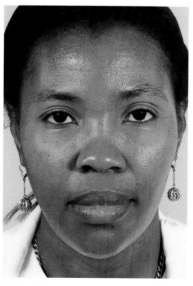

Color: Black
Reaction: Never burns, tans very easily

*Includes those of East Asian, Indian, and Oriental origin or those of African descent with lighter skin.

hyperpigmentation following resurfacing; however, these patients will be prone to premature skin aging if their lifestyles involve outdoor activities. Patients with Fitzpatrick types III and IV skin tan easily, suggesting that melanocytic proliferation will likely occur after skin resurfacing. This reaction needs to be controlled with a prepeel skin regimen if medium or deep resurfacing is planned, and sun avoidance and maintenance skin care are necessary after treatment to prevent blotchy hyperpigmentation.

Patients with Fitzpatrick types V and VI skin represent the greatest treatment challenge. Any resurfacing technique that penetrates the epidermal-dermal junction in these patients predisposes to hyperpigmentation even if an adequate prepeel regimen has been followed. The possibility of deep resurfacing producing loss of pigmentation must also be considered. In these types of individuals areas of skin may be tested in inconspicuous regions prior to performing full-face resurfacing, but these tests do not guarantee the final overall skin response. Fortunately patients with types V and VI skin rarely show clinical signs of photoaging.

Patients with light complexions who are less prone to facial pigment are excellent candidates for resurfacing because they tend to heal with uniform pigmentation. However, these patients are more susceptible to actinic damage and photoaging and commonly exhibit coarse and fine rhytides at an earlier age than patients with darker complexions.

Hair and eye color also help in evaluating a patient's response to chemical peeling or laser resurfacing. Skin evaluation is straightforward in patients with blond hair and blue eyes. Red-haired, freckled individuals are not prone to postpeel hyperpigmentation; however, they are more likely to develop hypopigmentation following deep resurfacing procedures. Some patients with dark hair and brown eyes have quite fair complexions, whereas other patients with fair complexions can appear dark from chronic sun exposure. Although hair and eye color is helpful, more precise information can be obtained by eliciting information regarding the response to actinic exposure. Examining the neck, chest, forearms, and protected skin overlying the breasts or inguinal region is helpful in determining the patient's natural complexion and its response to sun exposure.

All patients undergoing skin care treatment programs ranging from the dermatologic application of creams to superficial, medium, or deep resurfacing must be instructed in the use of sunscreens and sun avoidance. If the patient cannot or is unwilling to make the necessary lifestyle changes and commit to the use of sunscreens, the benefits of any treatment plan will be compromised.

Patients with significant actinic damage are commonly addicted to activities that involve sun exposure and may have difficulty in adapting to lifestyle changes. "Sun worshippers" with damaged skin are analogous to smokers who seek care for shortness of breath; common sense dictates that such patients can only obtain clinical improvement by changing their habits. Any clinical improvement gained by skin care treatment will be reversed when patients return to their previous lifestyle.

Clinical judgment is crucial to the treatment of dermal elastosis and its cosmetic effects. Patients with signs of early sun damage as exhibited by fine facial wrinkling who desire minimal peripeel morbidity can often be satisfactorily treated with daily skin care regimens and successive superficial peels performed at regular intervals. As dermal elastosis increases, a greater depth of dermal penetration is necessary and peripeel morbidity increases.

Most patients with photoaging complain of blotchy pigmentation or the presence of coarse and fine facial rhytides. Although numerous treatment options are available, proper selection of a treatment or a combination of treatment modalities will enhance the predictability of the result. In general our pretreatment program for facial hyperpigmentation begins with applications of Retin-A, hydroquinone, and glycolic or kojic acid preparations. Pigmentation from actinic exposure tends to be superficial in patients with types I and II skin, and these patients will commonly respond to daily skin care, sunscreens, and sun avoidance. Adjuvant treatment with superficial peeling agents is similarly successful in this subgroup of patients. In contrast, medium-depth peeling with trichloroacetic acid (TCA) is commonly required to treat hyperpigmentation in patients with types III and IV skin since the pigmentation is often localized to the dermis.

Fine facial rhytides will generally respond to either superficial or medium-depth peeling. Superficial peels will often need to be repeated frequently. Medium-depth TCA peels are particularly suited for fine wrinkles of the periorbital region, cheek, and forehead. Although coarse facial rhytides can be improved by medium-depth peels, this response is less predictable and of shorter longevity than that achieved by deep peeling agents or laser resurfacing.

Perioral rhytides are the most resistant to treatment, and our experience with medium-depth peeling has been disappointing; we believe that dermabrasion, laser resurfacing, or phenol peeling is indicated in these cases. In our opinion, regardless of the treatment modality, lower lip rhytides are more resistant to treatment than rhytides of the upper lip. Phenol produces the most consistent improvement in coarse perioral rhytides but also the greatest degree of hypopigmentation. This limits its usefulness in regional resurfacing. Laser resurfacing produces a predictable improvement in coarse perioral rhytides, although despite multiple passes with the laser, occasionally a single treatment will not remove all perioral lines in patients with severe actinic damage. A second laser treatment may be required in patients with coarse perioral rhytides, and the patient should be prepared for this possibility. Dermabrasion will usually eliminate most perioral rhytides and produces less hypopigmentation than phenol. In our opinion dermabrasion is as effective for perioral rhytides as laser resurfacing and produces a shorter duration of posttreatment erythema.

Patient Profiles

Classification of skin types is not a precise science. Hair color, eye color, and complexion must be evaluated. Actinic exposure may disguise the true skin color. Fair patients can appear to have dark complexions after chronic sun exposure. Since hair color obviously is affected by sun damage and hair tinting, it is often an unreliable guide.

Patients represent a wide spectrum of facial complexions and hair color. We have seen numerous examples of brunettes with fair complexions. Conversely, blond patients may exhibit significant pigmentation after sun exposure and may actually have darker complexions than their hair color suggests. These factors must be taken into consideration when evaluating skin type. In our opinion the best criterion for judging skin type is the patient's response to actinic exposure, that is, burns easily or tans readily in response to actinic exposure.

Skin Type I

Patients with type I skin tend to have either red or blond hair and eyes ranging from green to blue. Patients such as this will always burn on actinic exposure and therefore often avoid the sun. Thus these patients commonly exhibit facial rhytides as they age and rarely have pigmentary problems associated with actinic exposure, such as diffuse solar lentigines.

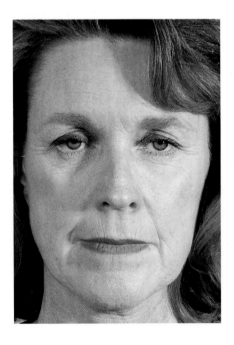

This patient is classified as having type I skin because of her fair complexion, green eyes, red hair, and reddish-colored eyebrows. She exhibits the gravitational effects of aging with dermal elastosis that is largely intrinsic in origin rather than secondary to actinic exposure. She shows little evidence of postinflammatory pigmentation and is ideal for any type of resurfacing procedure. Patients such as this are at risk for hypopigmentation following deep resurfacing and are poor candidates for regional phenol application because the line of demarcation between treated and untreated skin will be readily apparent.

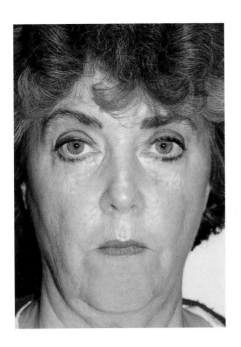

This woman has a fair complexion, red hair, and blue eyes. Although she rarely goes out in the sun, she has lived in the tropics all her life. Patients with type I skin are extraordinarily sensitive to even reflective sunlight. Even without prolonged actinic exposure and avoidance of activities such as sunbathing she shows a mosaic pattern of fine wrinkles. Patients with type I skin have virtually no protection from ultraviolet rays, and limited actinic exposure will lead to early facial rhytides. She will not be prone to postresurfacing pigmentation, but regional deep resurfacing may produce significant lightening in the area treated compared with adjacent untreated skin.

Skin Type II

Patients with type II skin will show intolerance to prolonged sun exposure, usually burning, but will also exhibit some tanning. Type II skin has limited protection from ultraviolet exposure, and both fine and coarse rhytides will develop if not properly protected. These patients do not tend to develop postresurfacing hyperpigmentation and are often ideal candidates for both medium-depth and deep peels as well as laser resurfacing.

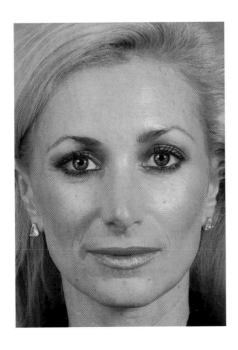

Because of sun sensitivity, patients with type II skin will commonly avoid the sun, as does this patient who has a fair complexion, blond hair, and blue eyes. Despite using sunscreens, mild actinic exposure has produced fine rhytides of her lower eyelids. Patients such as this are not prone to postresurfacing pigmentation. Because of the superficial nature of the fine lines on her lower lids, she is an ideal candidate for TCA peeling. Laser resurfacing will also provide long-term improvement but at the expense of a more prolonged posttreatment erythema.

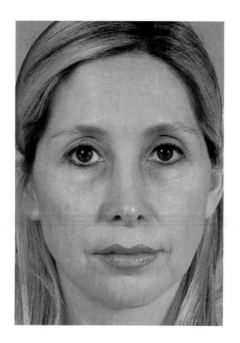

Despite her darker hair and brown eyes, this patient has type II skin. She tans easily, but avoidance of chronic actinic exposure has prevented premature wrinkling.

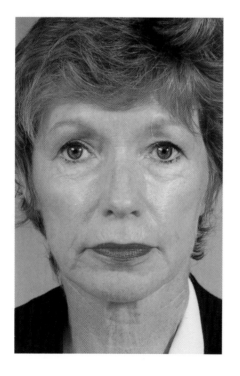

Some patients' skin types are difficult to categorize and may have features of different types. This woman has reddish blond hair, green eyes, and a fair complexion. Although she has protected her face from the sun, the pigmentation of her neck reveals the effect of minor actinic exposure. Note the leathery appearance of her neck in contrast to the younger, fresher appearance of her facial skin. Numerous treatment options are available in patients such as this. The lower eyelid rhytides will respond to medium-depth TCA peeling, although laser resurfacing will produce a better long-term result. Upper lid rhytides are best treated by either laser resurfacing or dermabrasion; however, dermabrasion in patients such as this may result in a slight hypopigmentation.

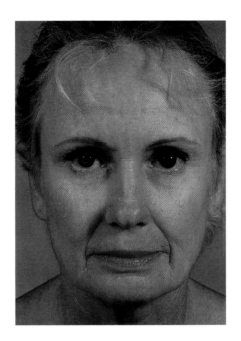

Not all patients with type II skin will avoid the sun and will continue to engage in activities such as tennis, golf, and boating despite their predilection to photoaging. This blond, blue-eyed patient with a fair complexion has a mottled pigmentation from chronic actinic exposure in association with rhytides of the lower eyelids and perioral region. Numerous treatment options are available for a patient with this complexion. Such patients will usually respond to medium-depth TCA peeling, which will ameliorate the mottled pigmentation and fine facial rhytides. For patients with coarse rhytides, more consistent results will be obtained with deeper resurfacing agents.

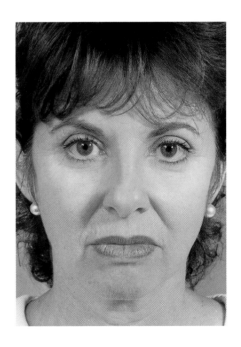

This patient exhibits characteristics of both types I and II skin. She has reddish hair, green eyes, and a fair complexion; however, her extremities indicate she tans in response to actinic exposure. Patients such as this show little tendency to posttreatment hyperpigmentation but are at risk for hypopigmentation if deep regional resurfacing agents are used.

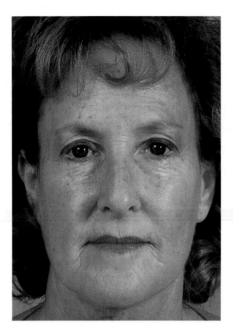 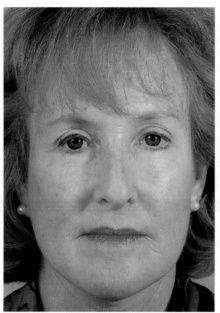

The classic changes associated with actinic exposure in patients with type II skin are seen here. This patient exhibits both coarse and fine facial rhytides as well as a mottled pigmentation and solar lentigines. A face lift was performed in conjunction with regional laser resurfacing of the lower eyelids and perioral region. Retin-A and hydroquinone were applied to the full face both before and after treatment. Facial mottling has resolved with a daily skin care regimen. Regional laser resurfacing has ameliorated her facial rhytides but left a slight degree of posttreatment hypopigmentation as compared with the adjacent untreated facial skin. Patients with types I and II skin are at greatest risk for hypopigmentation following use of deep resurfacing agents.

Skin Type III

Patients with type III skin readily tan, and with prolonged sun exposure they sometimes develop a mild sunburn. These patients usually have brown hair and brown eyes and show some tendency for hyperpigmentation following deep resurfacing procedures. Pretreatment with Retin-A and hydroquinone will help control hyperpigmentation in patients with this skin type.

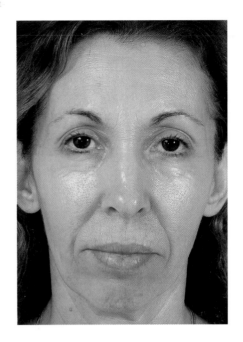

Some brown-haired individuals have fair complexions. This brunette has prototypical type III skin. Although the consequences of actinic exposure are minimal, there is some risk of posttreatment hyperpigmentation following laser resurfacing or chemical peel.

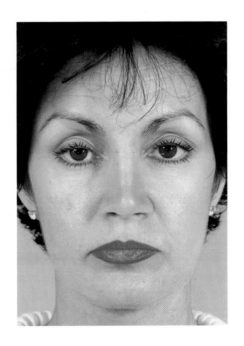

This patient is another example of a brunette, brown-eyed individual who has fair skin because of minimal actinic exposure. Despite her fair complexion, posttreatment hyperpigmentation is a real concern, and preoperative and posttreatment skin care regimens are essential to maintain consistent results.

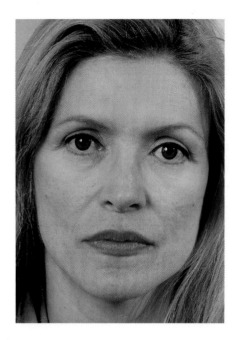

Some patients can be difficult to evaluate. This patient is of Hispanic origin but appears to have a fair complexion. Only her eye color gives her away. She lightens her hair, avoids the sun, uses sunscreens routinely, and follows a daily routine of Retin-A, hydroquinone, and glycolic acids. Her light complexion does not decrease her risk for hyperpigmentation should resurfacing procedures be used.

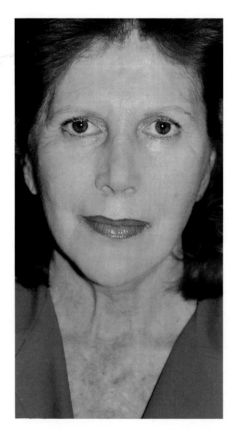

This patient has characteristics of both type II and type III skin. She has protected her face from the sun and shows little evidence of facial actinic exposure. The pigmentation she exhibits on her chest is typical of type II skin. Her facial pigmentation is uniform and rhytides are confined to the periorbital region. Patients such as this are ideal candidates for regional medium-depth TCA peels of the lower eyelids, although laser resurfacing may also be considered. Actinic damage of the neck and chest can be improved by pretreatment with Retin-A followed by a series of superficial peels with 20% to 30% TCA.

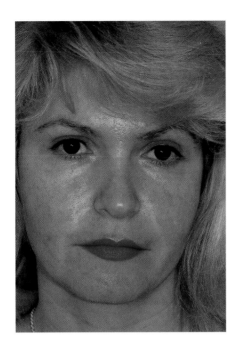

Using hair color as a guide to skin type may be misleading, especially since so many patients tint their hair. This patient appears to be a blond, yet her eyes and eyebrows are brown. Her blotchy pigmentation is secondary to chronic sun exposure. Wood's light fluorescence shows this pigmentation to be deep within the dermis. Prolonged pretreatment with Retin-A and hydroquinone followed by reticular dermal TCA peeling is a treatment option in patients such as this. To diminish the possibility of postinflammatory pigmentation, a prolonged skin care regimen as well as sun avoidance is required in these types of patients.

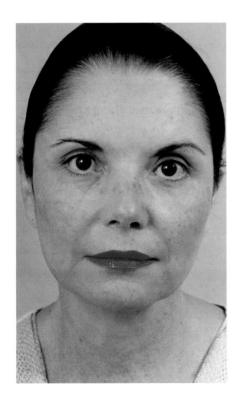

This woman has type III skin characteristics. She has dark brown hair and brown eyes but a light complexion. She has always been concerned about photoaging and has habitually avoided the sun and used sunscreens. The slight blotchy pigmentation of her neck and chest reveal her predilection to pigmentation with actinic exposure. Because of her diligence in avoiding the sun, a simple skin care regimen is all that is required.

Skin Type IV

Patients with type IV skin tend to have medium–dark complexions, dark brown to black hair, and brown to black eyes. These patients rapidly tan in response to sun exposure and rarely burn. Because of the significant pigmentation present in the epidermis, these patients are at high risk for hyperpigmentation after resurfacing. Prolonged pretreatment with Retin-A and hydroquinone is essential prior to medium-depth or deep resurfacing. These patients also require postresurfacing treatment with bleaching agents. Patients with type IV skin type are commonly of Mediterranean or Hispanic origin.

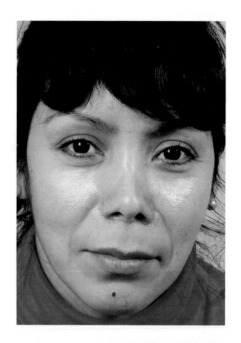

This Peruvian woman exhibits the characteristics of type IV skin. However, sun avoidance and the daily use of Retin-A and hydroquinone have lightened her skin. Her hair and eyes are dark brown and her skin is olive, but she shows no evidence of splotchy pigmentation because of her skin care routine and the use of sunscreens. Medium-depth TCA peeling can be safely performed in patients such as this as long as prepeel skin care is adequate.

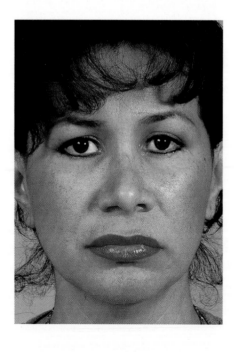

This 41-year-old patient from Guatemala has type IV skin and exhibits some evidence of actinic exposure. Her hair and eyes are dark brown and her complexion olive. Her splotchy pigmentation is more noticeable on her face than her chest. She is an excellent candidate for skin care routine consisting of Retin-A, hydroquinone, and glycolic acids. This in conjunction with sun avoidance and sunblocks should improve her blotchy pigmentation. Medium-depth TCA peeling can also be used after prolonged prepeel skin care to improve her appearance. Despite her age, she shows no evidence of fine or coarse facial wrinkling as is typical of patients with type IV skin.

Skin Type V

Patients with type V skin have dark complexions and usually black hair and dark eyes. These patients are commonly of Oriental, Indian, East Asian, or African descent. They tan deeply in response to sun and can exhibit profound splotchy pigmentation following a multitude of dermal injuries (trauma, acne, or viral infections). Skin resurfacing must be done judiciously in patients with type V skin. Pretreatment with Retin-A and hydroquinone is mandatory to prevent posttreatment hyperpigmentation. Consideration should be given to treating these patients with multiple superficial peeling agents and judging their response prior to undertaking deep resurfacing. With deep peeling, these patients are at risk not only for hyperpigmentation but also for uneven loss of pigment, which can produce a vitiligo-type appearance.

Patients with type V skin usually seek treatment for blotchy pigmentation. It is less risky to treat these patients with a daily skin care regimen and superficial peeling agents than to risk hyper- or hypopigmentation with deeper resurfacing methods. After proper preoperative preparation, medium-depth TCA peeling is a useful treatment modality to improve blotchy pigmentation in patients with this skin type.

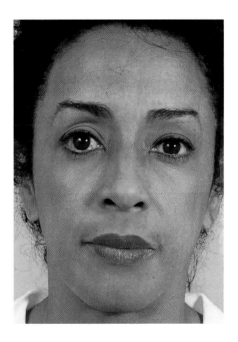

Patients of African descent with lighter skin exhibit the characteristics of type V skin, that is, black hair, dark eyes, and a dark complexion. This patient from the West Indies shows no evidence of chronic actinic exposure and her pigmentation is even. Despite approaching 50 years of age, she has essentially no facial rhytides and shows minimal evidence of the gravitational changes of aging or of dermal elastosis. The absence of weathered skin and the stigmata of early aging are typical in patients with type V skin. Because of the absence of photoaging, only daily skin care is required for most patients of this skin type.

Skin Type VI

Patients with type VI skin usually have a dark-brown complexion with black hair and dark eyes. These patients are typically of African descent. In response to sun exposure they will become deeply pigmented but never burn. The typical stigmata of photoaging are usually absent in patients with this skin type, although they can exhibit postinflammatory hyperpigmentation. Should resurfacing procedures be contemplated in patients with type VI skin, a prolonged pretreatment program is mandatory. Tendencies toward keloid formation and hypertrophic scarring should be elicited prior to contemplating a deep resurfacing treatment.

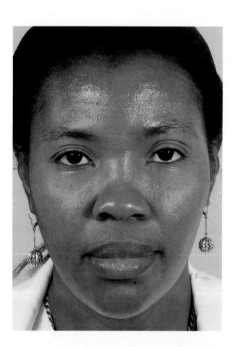

This 40-year-old woman is of African-American descent. Although she has been exposed to the sun most of her life, she shows no evidence of photoaging. The gravitational effects of aging are also slight compared with other patients of lighter skin types. The risk of posttreatment hyperpigmentation or loss of pigment following deep resurfacing is significant in patients such as this.

Skin Thickness and Texture

Skin thickness, pore size, and sebaceous secretions must be factored into the treatment plan. Skin thickness will vary from patient to patient and will influence the margin of safety during medium-depth or deep peels because the peeling agent will penetrate the reticular dermis more quickly in thin-skinned individuals.

Sebaceous secretions also influence treatment options. Patients with thick, oily skin will commonly respond well to a skin care program that suppresses oil production, and Retin-A and glycolic acids are usually well tolerated by these individuals. Residual oiliness of the skin prior to peeling makes the penetration of the peeling agent more difficult, and therefore patients with a significant degree of sebaceous activity require a more prolonged pretreatment regimen as well as more extensive degreasing at the time the peel is performed. Patients with chronic acne scarring commonly have thick, fibrotic skin that makes it more difficult for the peeling agent to penetrate adequately and requires aggressive pretreatment with Retin-A and hydroquinone prior to medium-depth peeling. In addition, multiple applications of TCA are generally necessary in these individuals to obtain adequate penetration.

Patients with thin, dry, atrophic skin represent a different clinical challenge. They tend to be more susceptible to sun damage than patients with thicker, oily skin. Many of these patients have significant photodamage associated with dermal atrophy and may tolerate pretreatment programs poorly that incorporate drying agents such as Retin-A or at times glycolic acids. The application of dermatologic agents must be graduated, and supplemental moisturizers are often required to ensure patient compliance. When these patients are adequately treated with Retin-A, peeling agents may penetrate the dermis rapidly. There is a smaller margin of safety in these individuals than in patients with thick, sebaceous skin. Most of the patients referred to us for hypertrophic scarring following resurfacing procedures have thin, dry skin. Consequently, resurfacing procedures must be performed with great care in this category of patients.

Patient Profiles

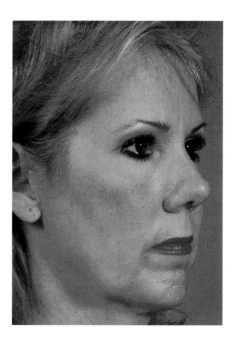

This patient has normal skin thickness and a normal degree of sebaceous activity. The effects of photoaging are minor, but gravitational influences on the facial soft tissues are more obvious. Since she exhibits little actinic damage, only daily skin care is necessary. If she exhibited advanced dermal elastosis, her complexion (type II), skin texture, and thickness would make her an ideal candidate for any skin resurfacing procedure.

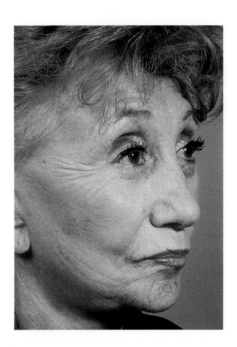

Patients with thin, dry skin often request facial resurfacing. The chronic effect of actinic exposure in fair patients with thin, dry skin is usually facial rhytides. Because of the lack of thickness of the dermis, resurfacing agents can penetrate quickly in these types of patients. Prepeel preparation with Retin-A before TCA peeling can lead to rapid penetration of the peel solution into the reticular dermis. Judging the depth of TCA penetration is essential in patients with this skin type. Similar considerations are warranted in laser resurfacing where the depth of resurfacing must be judged precisely.

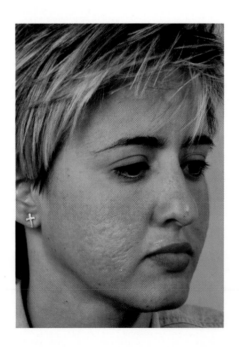

Patients with evidence of chronic acne scarring will usually have a thick, fibrotic dermis and oily skin. Deep resurfacing agents are usually required in patients with acne scarring. If TCA peeling is contemplated, pretreatment with Retin-A is essential to increase penetration of the peeling agent. The margin of safety in patients such as this who undergo TCA peeling is great because of the thickness of the dermis and its fibrotic consistency. Multiple applications of TCA are usually safe in such patients compared with patients with thin, dry skin. Because of the thick, fibrotic nature of the dermis, patients with acne scarring will usually show a more consistent response to treatment with dermabrasion or laser resurfacing than with medium-depth TCA peeling. There is little place for phenol peeling in the treatment of acne scars.

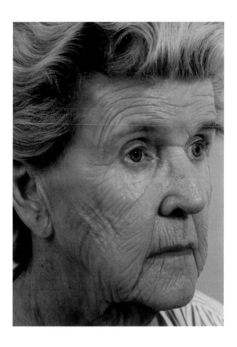

Chronic actinic exposure will ultimately lead to dermal atrophy and thinning of the skin. This woman has significant photodamage associated with coarse facial wrinkling and dry skin. Because of the severity of her wrinkling, superficial and medium-depth peels have little to offer. Her skin type makes her an ideal candidate for a full-face phenol peel or for full-face laser resurfacing.

DEGREE AND LEVEL OF PATHOLOGY

The two most common problems that prompt patients to request skin care treatment, skin peeling, or facial resurfacing are facial rhytides and problems with pigmentation. Both of these conditions are associated with excessive actinic exposure that leads to photodamage and are commonly associated with epithelial dysplasia. The degree of photodamage must be assessed before deciding on a treatment plan. It must be determined whether the pathologic condition is localized to the epidermis, the upper papillary dermis, or the mid to deep reticular dermis before judging the level of resurfacing required.

Dyschromias

Dyschromias represent alterations in pigmentation and clinically present as blotchy hyperpigmentation. Hyperpigmented lesions are typically seen in patients who have experienced prolonged actinic exposure. Fair-skinned individuals (usually with types I to III skin) present with a blotchy facial appearance from freckling, solar lentigines, nevi, and seborrheic keratoses. Prolonged sun exposure can also cause diffuse hyperpigmentation, which is essentially a coalescence of multiple solar lentigines, a condition termed melasma.

Postinflammatory pigmentation can follow any type of generalized skin irritation. This can be secondary to viral eruptions or drug allergies or a reaction to a topical stimulant that results in dermatitis. Postinflammatory pigmentation is frequently seen in patients with darker skin types (types III to IV). This is often a sequelae of acne scarring. Obviously these patients are at greatest risk for developing pigmentation disorders following skin resurfacing.

When evaluating a patient for dyschromia, it is important to determine the depth of the pathology. If the pigmentation is superficial, it is likely to respond to daily topical skin care and superficial peeling. If the pigmentation is localized to the papillary or upper reticular dermis, medium-depth or even deep skin resurfacing may be required.

We prefer to evaluate patients with dyschromias in a dark room using Wood's light to fluoresce the skin. Epidermal lesions fluoresce brightly under Wood's light, whereas dermal lesions appear darker and less distinct. If the dyschromia is within the dermis, epidermal peels will be ineffective.

Patients with postinflammatory pigmentation following facial resurfacing should be handled judiciously. Patients who develop postinflammatory pigmentation are pigment formers despite their underlying skin type, and restimulation will most likely produce further pigment formation. Prolonged use of topical creams (Retin-A, hydroquinone, and kojic acid) should be considered before further peeling is undertaken.

Once the level of pigmentation is ascertained, the key to achieving consistent results with resurfacing procedures is to first block the production of melanin through daily application of topical agents. If melanin resides within the dermis, deeper resurfacing can be performed only after epidermal melanin synthesis has been inhibited.

Facial Rhytides

Rhytides are the most common complaint of individuals seeking resurfacing. Superficial wrinkles often initially develop in the periorbital region (lower lid and crow's-feet areas). With aging, animation wrinkles develop and are evident in the perioral, glabellar, forehead, and anterior cheek areas. Gravitational changes influence the appearance and depth of these wrinkles.

Fine wrinkling responds to repeated superficial peels in conjunction with a daily skin care regimen. There is some evidence to suggest that repeated superficial epidermal peels influence the production of collagen formation in the dermis, producing a long-lasting improvement of fine rhytides. When wrinkling is deep or involves animation regions of the face, long-term results with superficial peeling agents are inconsistent and generally disappointing.

Although many patients are initially satisfied with the results of superficial peels and daily skin care, long-term improvement of facial rhytides requires deeper treatment with phenol peeling, dermabrasion, or laser resurfacing. Histologically, facial rhytides are associated with dermal elastosis that involves both the papillary and reticular dermis. Thus deep resurfacing agents that penetrate the reticular dermis must be used to stimulate neocollagen formation on healing. Because of the depth of treatment, increased patient morbidity and prolonged recovery must be expected.

Medium-depth TCA peels can improve the appearance of facial rhytides, especially repeated on a frequent basis to maintain the result. Because of the depth of penetration of medium-depth TCA peels and the lesser degree of neocollagen formation, the long-term improvement of coarse facial rhytides using TCA peels is inconsistent.

The physician must differentiate between wrinkles present in repose and those rhytides that are accentuated by animation. All forms of resurfacing are more successful in improving facial rhytides present at rest. Even after the most successful phenol peel patients will often exhibit facial rhytides during exaggerated animation. This is most obvious in the crow's-feet region, where orbicularis hypertrophy is not affected by skin resurfacing, and in the forehead, where concomitant brow ptosis remains as a stimulant to eyebrow elevation.

Gravitational Influences

Intrinsic and extrinsic aging of the skin is commonly associated with gravitational changes in the deeper facial soft tissues. The descent of facial fat and mimetic muscle is largely secondary to loss of support by the retaining ligaments of the face and usually accompanies dermal elastosis. Although facial resurfacing can improve appearance and restore dermal collagen, more youthful-appearing skin cannot counteract the gravitational changes affecting the deeper facial soft tissues. The patient must be apprised of this so she will not have unrealistic expectations.

Interestingly, some patients with rhytides along their cheeks can experience dramatic improvement with a face-lift procedure since wrinkles are less apparent following surgical tightening. We have had several patients who we thought would benefit from full-face resurfacing but they elected to have a face lift in conjunction with regional (perioral) peeling. Despite a more limited resurfacing approach in these patients, the results have often been dramatic, and commonly these patients have required either no further treatment or limited treatment with either superficial or medium-depth peels. Postoperative use of Retin-A, sunscreens, and sun avoidance is a useful adjunct in these types of patients.

Conversely, we have performed phenol peels and full-face laser resurfacing on patients we thought should undergo preliminary face lift and been surprised by an overall tightening of facial appearance associated with the neocollagen formation following deep peeling. Although deep resurfacing is not really a substitute for surgical tightening, the regeneration of new, elastic skin serves to significantly improve overall facial appearance.

FACIAL RESURFACING IN CONJUNCTION WITH SURGERY

Aesthetic surgery and full-face resurfacing are complementary procedures that we prefer to perform in stages. Although we perform regional resurfacing simultaneously with face lift, in general we delay full-face resurfacing until at least 3 months after the face-lift procedure. Similarly, we wait 3 months to resurface the lower eyelids following transcutaneous blepharoplasty. Transconjunctival blepharoplasty in association with laser resurfacing or TCA peeling of the lower eyelids can be safely performed simultaneously.

Skin that has been surgically undermined should rarely be subjected to simultaneous chemical peel, dermabrasion, or laser resurfacing. If a perioral peel or laser resurfacing is to be performed at the time of the face lift, we prefer to limit surgical undermining to a few centimeters lateral to the nasolabial fold. Resurfacing surgically insulted facial skin invites catastrophic hypertrophic scarring.

It will be difficult to camouflage the line of demarcation between treated facial skin and untreated cervical skin in patients with significant cervical obliquity in whom phenol peeling is planned. This problem must be carefully explained to the patient, and if both surgical intervention and chemical peeling for facial rhytides are planned, we prefer to perform the surgery first. Once the gravitational effects of aging have been corrected and the jawline-neck angle is sharp and distinct, chemical peeling will produce a less noticeable line of demarcation.

DEVELOPING A TREATMENT PLAN

Following assessment of the patient in terms of skin type, texture, and depth of pathology, a rational treatment plan can be developed. Several guidelines are used to formulate the treatment plan:

- *Patient morbidity:* The physician must determine how the anticipated therapy will affect a patient's lifestyle. Patients who have deep dermal pathology and cannot take time off from their daily activities are not candidates for deep resurfacing. Their lifestyle dictates that a daily skin care regimen and superficial peeling agents are appropriate. Effective patient education is required so that the patient understands that the results may be limited. Conversely, patients who elect to undergo deep resurfacing need to be advised about the length of time necessary before returning to work and social activities as well as the need for camouflaging makeup. For laser resurfacing or phenol peeling, patients usually require 2 weeks off work and the use of camouflaging cosmetics for 8 to 12 weeks. Often a compromise between the depth of pathology and the patient's lifestyle is required. Medium-depth TCA peeling is appropriate in patients with dermal pathology and lifestyle situations that limit the available time for recovery. After TCA peeling most patients can return to their daily activities with the use of minimal camouflaging makeup within 1 week.

- *Level of pathology:* Ascertaining the depth of pathology is key to formulating a logical treatment plan. Disorders localized to the epidermis do not require a phenol peel. Precision in determining the pathologic level and tailoring the resurfacing agent lend consistency and predictability to the procedure. In a similar fashion, experience teaches the physician how to read the resurfacing agent such that the peel, dermabrasion, or laser beam reaches the appropriate level in the dermis before treatment is terminated. This lends itself to predictable improvement while minimizing the possibility of posttreatment complications.

- *Risks associated with treatment:* Despite similar levels of pathology and skin types, not all patients are the same. Skin texture, dryness, associated systemic medical conditions, skin pretreatment, the previous use of Accutane, and a history of herpes simplex can greatly influence the postoperative course despite resurfacing to the appropriate level. Peels carried into the epidermis are associated with virtually no risk of scarring or pigmentary changes. Resurfacing taken into the reticular dermis always carries the risk of scarring, blotchy hyperpigmentation, or hypopigmentation. These factors must be taken into consideration when deciding whether a particular treatment agent and treatment level are appropriate. Phenol peeling produces significant hypopigmentation, limiting its applicability, especially if regional resurfacing is being considered. Medium-depth TCA peeling rarely produces permanent hypopigmentation but is associated with postinflammatory hyperpigmentation, especially in patients with type IV skin. This frequently occurs when skin pretreatment is inadequate. Although hypopigmentation is uncommon following laser resurfacing, it is seen in patients with types I and II skin with coarse rhytides who require resurfacing into the deep dermis. Often a compromise plan involving limited resurfacing in terms of depth of penetration will minimize the possibility of permanent pigmentary changes. Patient education regarding the possibility of a secondary procedure to correct residual rhytides is appropriate in this clinical situation.

Patient Consent Form for Facial Resurfacing

Physician _____

Name of patient _____

1. I hereby authorize Dr. _____ and associates to perform the facial resurfacing procedure(s) known as _____.

2. The procedure(s) and anticipated results have been explained to me, and I completely understand the nature and consequences of this treatment. The following points have been made clear:
   a. Although some improvement can be anticipated, the exact clinical change cannot be predicted. I acknowledge that no guarantee has been made regarding the condition of the complexion, skin pore size, elimination of wrinkles, or overall appearance.
   b. During resurfacing I will experience some discomfort and swelling. If dermabrasion, medium or deep chemical peeling, or laser therapy is performed, my face will be covered with a crust that will usually separate within 5 to 10 days.
   c. My skin will have a reddish appearance that may persist for several weeks if deeper peels are performed, and the skin at the juncture between treated and untreated areas may exhibit a difference in color, pigmentation, and texture.
   d. Alterations in pigmentation may occur in the treated areas.
   e. Small white bumps in the skin may persist for several months.
   f. In rare cases noticeable scarring can occur and cause visible disfiguration.

3. I recognize that unforeseen conditions may arise during the course of the procedure. I therefore authorize the above-named physician or his associates to perform any additional procedures that in his professional opinion are indicated.

4. If anesthesia is needed for the procedure(s), I consent to administration of such anesthetics as deemed advisable under the direction of my physician or his associate or a designated anesthesiologist.

5. I consent to be photographed before, during, and after treatment and understand that these photographs are the property of my physician and can be used for publication in the scientific literature or shown for scientific purposes.

6. I agree to return for follow-up visits as necessary and will cooperate fully with directions for posttreatment care regimens.

7. I have no known allergies except for _____.

CONSENT: By signing below I acknowledge that I have read the foregoing informed consent pertaining to facial resurfacing procedures and I believe the physician has adequately informed me of the risks of said procedures, anticipated results, and alternative methods of treatment.

Date _____ Time _____

Patient's signature _____

Witness _____

Signature of parent or guardian if patient is a minor _____

Patient Profiles: Clinical Decision Making

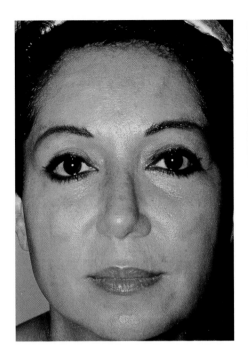 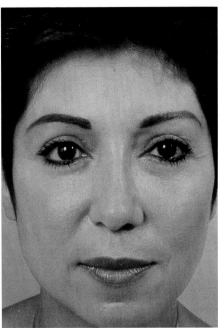

Skin Type & Complexion: Type IV

Thickness & Texture: Medium thickness, oily skin

Level & Type of Pathology: Dyschromia localized to epidermis and papillary dermis following prolonged sun exposure

Risks: Postinflammatory hyperpigmentation following resurfacing

Options & Treatment: This Hispanic patient was very compliant in terms of further sun avoidance and the use of Retin-A and hydroquinone on a daily basis. Because of the success of the pretreatment skin regimen, a single medium-depth 35% TCA peel was performed. In patients with type IV skin the risk of posttreatment hyperpigmentation is substantial, making prolonged pretreatment with hydroquinone to suppress epidermal melanocytes essential. In our opinion phenol peeling would be inappropriate in this patient because of the risks of hypopigmentation or severe postinflammatory hyperpigmentation. Also the morbidity of deep resurfacing is inappropriate in view of the superficial depth of the pathology in the dermis.

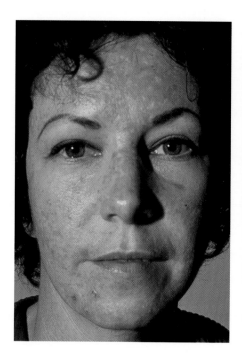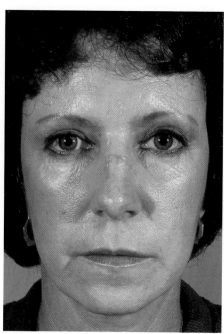

Skin Type & Complexion: Type III

Thickness & Texture: Medium thickness, oily skin

Level & Type of Pathology: Dyschromia localized to epidermis and papillary dermis following repeated bouts of adolescent acne

Risks: Postinflammatory hyperpigmentation following resurfacing

Options & Treatment: This 25-year-old woman developed blotchy hyperpigmentation following repeated bouts of adolescent acne. We treated her years ago when treatment options were limited. She is shown 10 years after a full-face phenol peel that corrected the dyschromia. The scar on her nose is not related to the peel.

   Today phenol would not be our first choice. Patients with this type of problem typically respond to prolonged pretreatment with Retin-A, hydroquinone, kojic acid, and sunscreens. Medium-depth TCA peeling following adequate pretreatment would most likely have improved her appearance with less postoperative morbidity or the risk of posttreatment hypopigmentation.

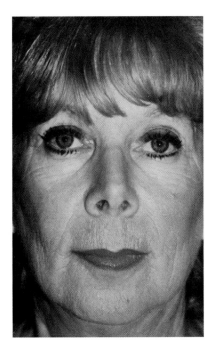 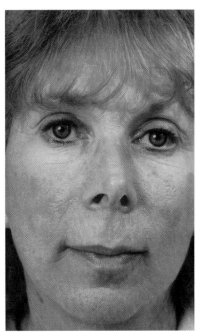

Skin Type & Complexion: Type II

Thickness & Texture: Medium to thin thickness, dry skin

Level & Type of Pathology: Fine and coarse facial rhytides localized to papillary and reticular dermis and gravitational changes of aging

Risks: Hypopigmentation following resurfacing

Options & Treatment: This 62-year-old patient shows the effect of actinic exposure on type II skin. She exhibits evidence of coarse and fine wrinkling as well as the gravitational influences of aging. Her initial treatment consisted of upper and lower blepharoplasty, rhytidectomy, and upper lip dermabrasion. She is shown following a medium-depth 35% TCA peel performed 8 months after surgery. Note that the cheek rhytides appear improved, which is largely the result of the face-lift procedure. The lower eyelid rhytides have responded to the lower lid blepharoplasty and subsequent TCA peel. Upper lip dermabrasion has improved the perioral lines, producing only minor color changes.

Alternative resurfacing options in this patient would include perioral lower eyelid laser resurfacing. Regional phenol peeling tends to produce significant hypopigmentation in patients such as this and is not recommended.

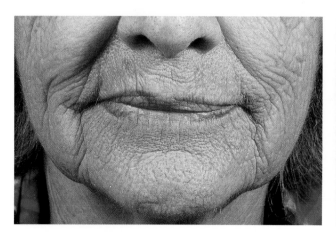 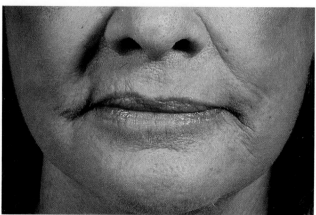

Skin Type & Complexion: Type II

Thickness & Texture: Medium thickness, dry skin

Level & Type of Pathology: Fine and coarse rhytides

Risks: Hypopigmentation following resurfacing

Options & Treatment: This patient demonstrates the effects of prolonged sun exposure. Poor skin quality as opposed to gravitational influences of aging is the culprit. She is shown following full-face laser resurfacing. Note the improvement of facial wrinkling without severe hypopigmentation. This represents one of the greatest advantages of laser resurfacing. Although phenol peeling or dermabrasion could have been used in this patient, the pigmentary changes would have been more severe. The skin appears to be tighter following resurfacing, demonstrating the elasticity of rejuvenated facial skin associated with dermal neocollagen formation.

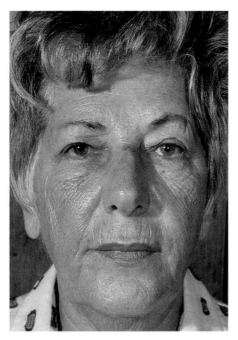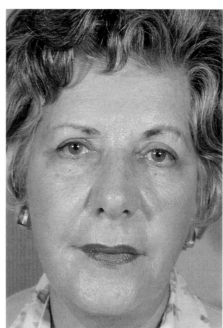

Skin Type & Complexion: Type II

Thickness & Texture: Medium thickness, dry skin

Level & Type of Pathology: Fine and coarse facial rhytides and gravitational influences of aging

Risks: Hypopigmentation and possible hypertrophic scarring following deep resurfacing

Options & Treatment: This patient also exemplifies the effects of actinic exposure on type II skin. Her skin is deeply tanned and she has both coarse and fine facial rhytides. The gravitational effects of aging are significant despite her age, giving her the appearance of an elderly woman. This patient initially had an upper and lower blepharoplasty and rhytidectomy to correct the gravitational changes of aging. Three months following surgery she had a full-face phenol peel. She is shown 6 months after the chemical peel.

Patients such as this are best treated with a combination of surgery and resurfacing. Resurfacing alone will not correct facial laxity; nor will surgery alone improve the weathered appearance of her skin. Today, we would most likely use full-face laser resurfacing rather than phenol peeling to treat this patient to avoid hypopigmentation postoperatively. The risk of laser resurfacing in the treatment of coarse rhytides such as these is that the laser penetration must extend well into the reticular dermis. The risk of hypertrophic scarring from multiple passes of the laser must be considered. Medium-depth TCA peeling is inappropriate for this level of pathology and would provide insignificant long-term improvement.

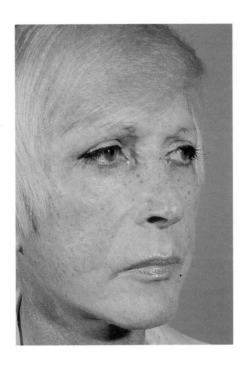

Skin Type & Complexion: Type I

Thickness & Texture: Medium thickness, dry skin

Level & Type of Pathology: Dyschromia localized to the epidermis and papillary dermis and fine facial wrinkles as a result of sun exposure

Risks: Severe hypopigmentation following resurfacing

Options & Treatment: As a tennis player, this 44-year-old patient has suffered significant sun damage. Her moderate tan disguises how fair she really is. Inspection of nonexposed parts of her body shows that she has characteristics of type I skin. Patients such as this are at risk for hypopigmentation with deep resurfacing. Dyschromias in these patients are usually superficial and respond to daily skin care regimens and sun avoidance. Superficial peeling as well as medium-depth TCA peels are useful adjuncts in improving the appearance in these types of patients. Unfortunately, this patient underwent a regional phenol peel and developed severe hypopigmentation with an obvious line of demarcation between treated and untreated skin. Dermabrasion could have been used, but the risk of hypopigmentation would have been the same. Although hypopigmentation following laser resurfacing is less common, patients such as this are not without risk. In retrospect, because this patient's pathology was limited to the superficial dermis, a deep resurfacing agent should not have been used.

CONCLUDING THOUGHTS

Aesthetic surgery is a visual art in which facial beauty must be interpreted differently for each patient. Individualization of treatment planning is requisite to obtaining consistently good results. No one procedure offers pat answers. Facial skin resurfacing, like all aesthetic surgery of the face, requires proper patient evaluation. In addition to assessment of the physical characteristics of facial skin, proper patient communication and rapport are essential. Understanding what motivates patients to seek medical treatment and how disturbed they are by their particular problem is an important ingredient in clinical decision making. Only through an understanding of the patient's needs, lifestyle, and ultimate objectives can the physician and patient achieve their mutual goals.

REFERENCES

Baker TJ, Gordon HL, Stuzin JM. Chemical peeling (phenol and trichloroacetic acid) and dermabrasion. In Surgical Rejuvenation of the Face, 2nd ed. St. Louis: Mosby, 1996, p 45.

Brody HJ. Chemical Peeling. St. Louis: Mosby–Year Book, 1992.

Fitzpatrick TB. The validity and practicality of sun-reactive skin types I through VI. Arch Dermatol 124:869, 1988.

Gilchrest BA, Szabo G, Flynn E, Goldwyn RM. Chronologic and actinically induced aging in human facial skin. J Invest Dermatol 80:815, 1983.

Kligman AM, Lauker RM. Cutaneous aging: The difference between intrinsic aging and photoaging. J Cutan Aging Cosmet Dermatol 1:5, 1988.

Matarasso SL, Glogau RG. Chemical face peels. Dermatol Clin 9:131, 1991.

Rubin MG. Manual of Chemical Peels, Superficial and Medium Depth. Philadelphia: JB Lippincott, 1995.

Stuzin JM, Baker TJ, Gordon HL. Treatment of photoaging: Facial chemical peeling (phenol and trichloroacetic acid) and dermabrasion. Clin Plast Surg 20:9, 1993.

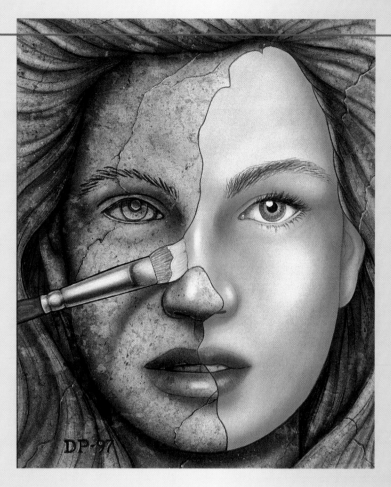

Skin Care Agents and Superficial Peels

The numerous products commercially available for skin rejuvenation are a reflection of our culture's emphasis on preserving a youthful appearance. In the past decade the distinction between common beauty products and prescription skin care agents has become blurred. Cosmetic companies now offer products in more dilute concentrations that were previously available only by prescription. Similarly, physician-dispensed products now include a variety of agents that closely resemble cosmetics. The commercial and medical markets have become inundated with products extolling the virtues of their creams and emollients. The physician must sort through these claims and products carefully to be able to recommend preparations whose efficacy is based on scientific evidence and confirmed by clinical trial.

Cleansers, moisturizers, and sunscreens are basic skin care agents designed for daily use. These maintenance products keep pores clean, moisturize skin, and offer protection from the sun. The next line of creams to enhance actinically damaged skin includes keratolytic agents (alpha hydroxy acids) that improve skin texture and creams (hydroquinone and kojic acid) that inhibit melanocyte function and ameliorate facial dyschromia. Retin-A, which has long been used to treat acne, is commonly used in conjunction with other creams to enhance their pharmacologic effect. Skin care agents not only represent a coordinated skin care routine for daily maintenance but are also used as a pretreatment regimen prior to medium-depth or deep resurfacing.

Daily skin care agents in conjunction with appropriately timed superficial peels will improve sun-damaged skin with only minimal posttreatment morbidity. Superficial peels using Jessner's solution, high-concentration glycolic acid, and low-concentration trichloroacetic acid are ideally suited for treating pathologic conditions situated superficially within the skin, specifically the epidermis. These agents can predictably enhance skin texture and ameliorate disorders of facial pigmentation when the pigment is localized to the basement membrane. Although transient improvement of fine rhytides is possible, frequent retreatment is required to maintain the result. Sun protection, sun avoidance, a compliant patient, and regular monitoring of the skin care routine are key to consistency and longevity of results.

SKIN CARE AGENTS

Improving actinically damaged skin begins with a daily skin care program. This routine is individualized and must become a long-term commitment to be effective. The basic components of any program are cleansers, moisturizers, sunscreens, Retin-A, alpha hydroxy acids, and hydroquinones. Other agents commonly used to treat photoaged skin include kojic acid and Cellex-C. After a patient has followed a skin care program for 6 to 8 weeks, supplemental peels may also be performed if necessary to accelerate skin rejuvenation.

A skin care program is prescribed after a detailed examination of the skin (see Chapter 3). This approach will determine the specific needs of each patient and will frequently identify associated skin pathologies. The final regimen should be simple and inexpensive to ensure patient compliance.

Cleansers

Cleansers are an essential component of any skin care routine. These products are designed to keep the skin's surface free of oils, dirt, and surface exfoliants. All pretreatment products are more effective when applied to a clean, oil-free surface. Accordingly, patients should scrub their faces with mild soap and water prior to the application of any skin care product.

Moisturizers

Moisturizers appear to have two effects. They import oils directly into the stratum corneum, helping to smooth the skin's texture and appearance. They also slow water evaporation from the skin's surface by coating the skin with an oily layer, thereby preventing the desiccation of the outer layers of the epidermis and reducing keratin buildup. Use of these skin agents is individualized according to the oiliness or dryness of the patient's skin, with care taken to avoid products that are comedogenic.

Before advising a patient about moisturizers we inquire about the patient's daily routine. If Retin-A and lower concentrations of alpha hydroxy acids are being used, patients will tend to have dry facial skin. Moisturizers will help ameliorate these untoward side effects. If the patient is not using a moisturizer or is using one that is not effective and the skin appears dry and flaky, the skin care routine is modified accordingly. Patients will respond differently to various products, and efficacy is a function of patient compliance and preference.

Sunscreens

It is critical that all patients undergoing prepeel treatment use sunscreens. Photoaged skin has the capacity to repair itself to some degree if protected from sun. Retinoids and alpha hydroxy acids sensitize the skin to sun exposure and make the patient more vulnerable to ultraviolet (UV) burning and damage. We counsel our patients about the detrimental effects of UV light and the need to protect themselves from sun exposure. The daily use of sunscreens is an important aspect of treatment. Just a few minutes of UV exposure can reverse the results of months of skin preparation and peels.

Sunscreens work synergistically with hydroquinone and Retin-A to protect against UV-induced melanocytic hypertrophy in patients who are undergoing peeling for hyperpigmentation. We recommend using sunscreens that block not only UVB light but also UVA light such as Shade-UVA. The UVA wavelength is the band of light that stimulates melanocytic proliferation and produces facial rhytides. In patients who suffer from pigmentation disorders it is especially important to block this penetrating band of UV light. We prefer clear formula sunscreens that have a sun protection factor (SPF) of 15 or higher, have a waterproof base, and are relatively inexpensive. If a patient is allergic to para-aminobenzoic acid, sunscreens that do not contain this chemical should be substituted. In conjunction with the UVA blocking sunscreens, we suggest that our patients use creams containing micronized titanium dioxide such as Neutrogena Chemical Free. These types of sunscreens mechanically block all bands of UV light and work synergistically with chemical blocking sunscreens. Patients should apply waterproof sunscreens 30 minutes before engaging in swimming or vigorous outdoor activities and reapply them frequently.

Retin-A Cream

Tretinoin (Retin-A), the *all-trans*-retinoic acid derivative of vitamin A, is the mainstay of daily skin care because it can reverse the histologic and clinical damage resulting from actinic exposure. Retin-A predominantly affects the epidermis, although dermal changes can occur with prolonged application. Its epidermal effects (thinning of the stratum corneum and melanocyte suppression) make it an ideal pretreatment agent for resurfacing procedures. Retin-A enhances penetration of the peeling solutions and speeds reepithelialization time.

The clinical and histologic effects of Retin-A are well documented in reversing photoaging. The effects of Retin-A are mediated by a specific cellular binding protein through differential gene modulation. Clinical changes begin 6 to 12 weeks after initiation of treatment and the benefits may not be fully realized for 6 to 12 months. The skin will exhibit a smoother texture, a pink healthy glow, and a more homogeneous pigmentation. Histologically, the epidermis appears less dysplastic with fewer actinic keratoses and a more uniform distribution of melanin granules. The cellular portion of the epidermis becomes thicker as vertical polarity returns with epidermal maturation, whereas the stratum corneum becomes thinner and more permeable. The dermal changes include increased angiogenesis with new collagen synthesis.

The initial pretreatment plan begins with applications of 0.1% Retin-A. Because of the potential irritant effects associated with Retin-A and possible problems with patient compliance should retinoid dermatitis (xerosis and erythema) develop, we initially prescribe a small amount of the cream and gradually increase the frequency and volume of application as tolerated. The majority of patients will initially experience a transient dermatitis, but this generally abates within 2 to 3 weeks. We instruct patients to apply a small amount of cream to the entire face at bedtime (usually a volume comparable to a pea or small grape). Most patients can tolerate this concentration of Retin-A every other night. Patients tend not to apply the Retin-A uniformly to the face, concentrating on those areas of their complexion that they find most troubling, such as areas of facial wrinkling. Since spotty application of Retin-A will result in uneven uptake of the peeling solution, we stress uniform application over the face, including the lower lid and crow's-feet areas, reaching up to the hairline and extending to the preauricular area of the cheeks. If the neck or chest is to be

Patient Instructions for Use of Retin-A

1. Wash your face thoroughly. First apply a small amount of Retin-A (about the size of a pea) uniformly to the entire face except for the corners of the mouth, corners of the nose, and the eyelid margins every other night.
2. Allow the Retin-A to dry before applying a moisturizer to the face.
3. In the morning wash your face, apply a sunscreen (SPF No. 19), and then use a moisturizer.
4. If your skin becomes irritated, use a smaller volume of Retin-A every third or fourth night. If you continue to experience problems with this reduced regimen, stop using the cream and call your physician.
5. After you are able to tolerate the cream, increase the volume and apply nightly.

peeled, Retin-A is applied to these areas as well. Patients may be reevaluated at 2- to 3-week intervals to assess compliance, monitor clinical improvement, and fine-tune the skin care regimen.

If the skin becomes irritated, we try to discourage the patient from discontinuing the medication but rather suggest using a smaller amount and applying the cream every third or fourth night until more frequent applications can be tolerated. Alternatively, the concentration of Retin-A cream can be reduced to 0.05% or less. If patients cannot tolerate even a low-dose Retin-A routine, we usually supplement the Retin-A application with hydrocortisone cream. In addition, moisturizers may help ameliorate some of these undesirable responses. If the Retin-A continues to irritate the patient's skin and inhibits satisfactory patient compliance, we suggest eliminating Retin-A and substituting a glycolic acid preparation ranging from 10% to 14% in concentration.

After the patient can tolerate the application of Retin-A every other night (usually in 2 to 4 weeks), we increase the frequency of application to every night. Once daily application is tolerated, the concentration and volume of Retin-A can be increased as desired. Patients are instructed that Retin-A causes increased photosensitivity, mandating the use of sunscreens. For patients with dry skin, 0.05% Renova is an alternative. The retinoic acid in this formulation is not as drying as Retin-A (which is prescribed for acne) and is commonly better tolerated as a daily skin care agent.

Hydroquinone Cream

Hydroquinone cream is used to prepare the skin for chemical peels, to maintain uniform pigmentation after peeling, and to prevent postpeel hyperpigmentation. It can also be used in conjunction with Retin-A, alpha hydroxy acid, or kojic acid for the treatment of superficial dyschromias. This topically applied compound causes reversible depigmentation. It inhibits enzymatic oxidation of tyrosine 3,4-dihydroxyphenylalanine (dopa) and helps suppress melanin production in the basal epidermis. Because it prevents only the formation of new melanin, it will take several weeks before its clinical effects are noticeable.

In patients with Fitzpatrick types III to V skin we routinely add hydroquinone to the prepeel regimen. The effectiveness of hydroquinone is enhanced by the simultaneous use of Retin-A, which increases the penetration, working synergistically to suppress melanocytic metabolism.

Hydroquinone cream is applied simultaneously with Retin-A. Because it can be irritating to the skin, it is initially used every other night and the frequency increased as tolerated. We generally use Solaquin Forte (ICN Pharmaceuticals), which contains both 4% hydroquinone and an SPF 15 sunscreen. In patients with severe hyperpigmentation disorders or those with dark complexions, hydroquinone may be used twice daily, both at night with Retin-A and in the morning as a solitary agent. When used in conjunction with Retin-A, we have the patient mix an equal amount of the two agents together and then apply evenly to the facial skin. Recently several companies have produced combination creams containing 4% hydroquinones and Retin-A with or without various other additives (sunscreens, 1% hydrocortisone, and kojic acid) that have simplified the daily routine.

RESULTS

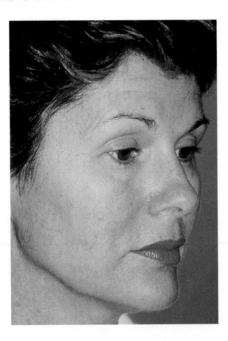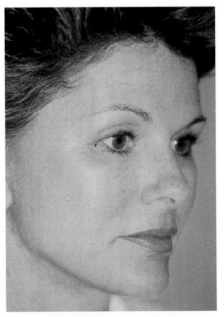

This patient with Fitzpatrick type II skin exhibits mild photoaging and fine facial rhytides. She had a face lift and then implemented a skin care regimen consisting of sunscreens and Retin-A. The improved pigmentation and skin texture are attributable to her skin care program and sun avoidance.

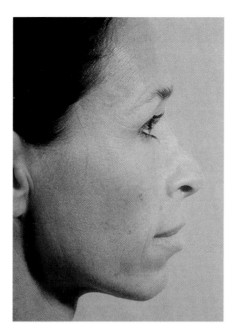 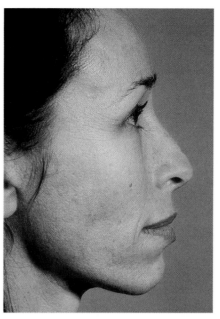

This patient with Fitzpatrick type II skin shows the effects of prolonged sun exposure and the results that can be achieved with a daily regimen of Retin-A and hydroquinone combined with sun avoidance and sunscreens.

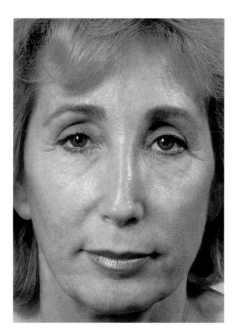 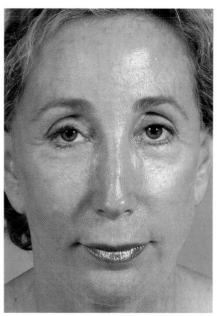

The fine facial rhytides and blotchy pigmentation in this woman with Fitzpatrick type II skin were ameliorated by a skin care routine consisting of Retin-A, glycolic acids, and hydroquinone. She is shown 4 years after initiating this regimen.

Kojic Acid

Kojic acid is commonly used as a bleaching agent. Like hydroquinone, it blocks the conversion of tyrosine to L-dopa, thereby preventing the formation of new melanin. It takes one to two cell cycles (45 to 90 days) for the effect of this agent to be evident because it has no effect on existing melanin. Kojic acid is available as a 2% to 3% gel or in combination with hydroquinones and other active agents such as Retin-A, alpha hydroxy acids, and corticosteroids. This compound is an excellent alternative for patients with pigmentary problems who cannot tolerate Retin-A, as is often the case immediately following laser resurfacing when the skin is extremely sensitive. Patients with severe dyschromias will commonly respond to combined Retin-A and hydroquinone applied at night and a combination of kojic acid and hydroquinone applied in the morning.

Cellex-C

A new product gaining popularity among physicians and patients is Cellex-C, a stable 10% aqueous solution of vitamin C that can be applied topically and absorbed directly by the skin. The skin is able to absorb more than 20 times the amount of nonionized ascorbic acid than the intestinal tract. Once the targeted skin has absorbed Cellex-C, it cannot be removed by washing or rubbing. The effects of Cellex-C are basically twofold. First, as an antioxidant, it is capable of neutralizing oxygen free radicals generated by UV light and inflammation. Second, Cellex-C is reported to stimulate new collagen formation. Laboratory data are more plentiful than clinical data at this time.

Cellex-C is applied uniformly to the entire facial skin one to two times daily. The full clinical effect may not be seen for up to 6 months, although initial improvement is frequently evident in 1 to 2 weeks. Fine facial rhytides appear less obvious and the texture of the facial skin is smoother. Cellex-C seems to cause less irritation and drying of the skin than Retin-A and glycolic acids and is usually well tolerated by patients. However, this product is very expensive. It is our impression that clinical improvement can be observed more rapidly with Cellex-C than with the glycolic acids. This may be a consequence of epidermal hydration following its application. The clinical effects of Cellex-C are reversed once its use is discontinued.

SUPERFICIAL CHEMICAL PEELING AGENTS

Superficial peeling agents are used to treat pathologic conditions localized to the epidermis and the most superficial portions of the dermis. These agents are effective for treating actinic keratoses, fine facial wrinkles, superficial dyschromias, and the changes associated with mild actinic damage. Generally a series of several peels is performed over weeks or months.

Superficial peels have several advantages over deeper peels. They are ideal for patients whose lifestyles preclude a longer recovery time associated with the deeper resurfacing modalities. Patients can return to work the same day the peel is performed. Since there is no hypopigmentation associated with these treatments, there is no line of demarcation between treated and untreated areas. Superficial agents are more "patient friendly"; they are not painful, are not associated with prolonged or complicated wound care, and are generally safe and rarely associated with complications and adverse outcomes.

Indications

Ideal candidates for superficial peels are patients in their thirties or forties who complain of spotty pigmentation and dull, "tired" skin. These patients exhibit pigmentary irregularities, fine rhytides, and actinic keratoses. The goal of treatment is to produce a healthier, more vibrant appearance with the elimination of pigmentary irregularities. After a superficial peel the skin appears to glow and fine rhytides are improved. These peels also produce a smoother skin texture, which enhances the result. Patients, however, must be selected carefully and educated realistically; repeated treatments are often required to achieve the desired appearance. These individuals must have the motivation and lifestyle that will permit them to adhere to a daily skin care program.

The pathologic condition treated should be restricted primarily to the epidermis, that is, within the range of penetration of the selected peeling agent. Examination using Wood's light will help identify those patients who may respond favorably to a superficial peeling agent. Pigmentary abnormalities limited to the epidermis become enhanced under Wood's lamp illumination and should improve following superficial peeling and daily skin care. Superficial peeling is not appropriate for patients with coarse facial rhytides. Deeper dyschromias exhibit minimal enhancement under Wood's lamp illumination and will require more aggressive therapies (medium-depth or deep resurfacing).

A number of superficial peeling agents are available. Some of the most frequently used compounds include Jessner's solution, alpha hydroxy acids, 10% to 25% trichloroacetic acid (TCA), and 50% salicylic acid.

Jessner's Solution

Jessner's solution (formulated by Dr. Max Jessner) has been in clinical use for over a century. The formula is as follows:

Resorcinol	14 gm
Salicylic acid	14 gm
Lactic acid (85%)	14 gm
Ethanol (95%)	100 ml

Jessner's solution produces keratolysis and protein coagulation. It removes the stratum corneum and keratocoagulates significant portions of the epidermis. Repeated applications will result in deeper penetration. Its mechanism of action appears to be lysis of bridges between keratinocytes. It may be used as a peeling agent alone or in conjunction with a TCA peel to enhance TCA penetration. The solution is stored in a closed amber glass bottle due to its sensitivity to air and light. It has a distinct medicinal aroma and will turn pink on exposure to the air.

Technique, Postpeel Care, and Complications

The procedure is performed in an outpatient setting without sedation or analgesia. The patient's skin is pretreated with Retin-A and hydroquinones to increase the effectiveness of Jessner's solution. The skin is cleansed and vigorously degreased with alcohol or acetone. Gauze sponges moistened with Jessner's solution are used for application. The solution can be carried into the eyebrows and anterior hairline and inferiorly 2 to 3 cm below the mandibular margin. If other pathologic conditions are present on the neck, anterior chest, or hands, these regions may be treated in a similar fashion. Unlike glycolic acid, neutralization with water or alkaline solutions is not necessary.

The depth of penetration and the end point of the peel are determined by the clinical appearance of the skin. A single, even application in well-prepared skin produces mild erythema, minimal stinging or tingling that resolves in 5 to 10 minutes, and flaking that lasts only 1 or 2 days. Two to three applications of the solution produce a deeper level of peeling typified by moderate stinging lasting up to 30 minutes and mild erythema. Occasionally isolated regions of light frost can be seen. In these cases the skin appears slightly sunburned for several days and may show signs of flaking for 3 or 4 days. More than three applications of solution will produce a deep Jessner peel. The depth of peel is characterized by bright erythema and splotchy regions of light frost associated with additional patient discomfort. Although no open wounds are produced, peeling and flaking may persist for a week or more.

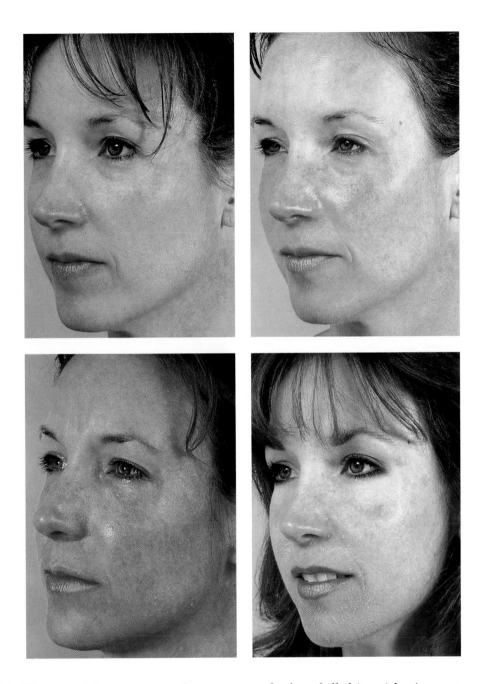

This 38-year-old woman sought treatment for her dull skin with pigmentary ir-regularities. She is shown 2 minutes following the application of a single layer of Jessner's solution. The regions around the mouth and below the eyes demonstrate deeper uptake of Jessner's solution secondary to pretreatment of these areas with Retin-A. Four minutes following application of two layers of Jessner's solution there is a uniform pink-red background with splotchy areas of light frosting. Superficial flaking resulting from epidermal desquamation is evident 3 days after Jessner's peeling.

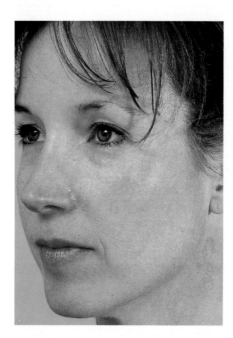 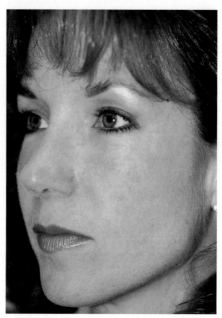

Healing is complete 2 weeks after peeling. The skin is smoother, healthier, and less blotchy. A maintenance skin care routine, sunscreens, and sun avoidance will help prolong this result.

Postpeel care is straightforward. A bland moisturizer is applied three to four times a day. This soothes the skin and limits the severity and visibility of the flaking. Sunscreens are mandatory since the skin's protective outer layer is removed, making it more vulnerable to the effects of UV light. Retin-A and preparations containing alpha hydroxy acids are usually discontinued for a week. Makeup may be applied over the moisturizer as desired.

Jessner's peels may be repeated at 1- to 3-week intervals depending on the patient's tolerance and the depth of the previous peel. The number of peels required is determined by the clinical response. Superficial pathologies may exhibit immediate improvement, whereas deeper problems frequently require repeated applications. Pathologic conditions that do not respond after several peels may require more aggressive therapies.

Jessner's solution is also used as a prepeel treatment prior to application of 35% TCA solution. Prepeel application disrupts the normally protective epidermis and allows a deeper, more uniform peel. Use of Jessner's solution prior to TCA application is indicated for patients with thick skin, those who have more severe actinic damage, and those in whom inadequate skin preparation is suspected. Once the skin is prepared and cleansed, one or several coats of Jessner's solution are applied to the facial skin until mild to moderate erythema is noted. Thicker, more actinically damaged skin may require several coats of Jessner's solution prior to the TCA peel. Pretreatment with Jessner's solution is usually unnecessary for thinner, less damaged skin.

Complications are unlikely because Jessner's peel has limited penetration. Prolonged erythema and occasional hyperpigmentation occur. Erythema is self-limiting and hyperpigmentation is a sequela of unprotected early UV exposure. Allergic reactions to the resorcinol are exceedingly rare in all large reports. Resorcinol and particularly salicylic acid both have the potential for systemic toxicity. This small risk can be minimized by avoiding application to large surface areas or multiple areas at the same time.

Alpha Hydroxy Acids

Alpha hydroxy acids (AHAs) are naturally occurring acids with carbon chains of variable lengths and a terminal carboxyl group. This group of chemicals includes glycolic, lactic, citric, malic, and tartaric acids. AHAs appear to exert their clinical effects by reducing corneocytic cohesion. This results in thinning of the stratum corneum, which improves surface texture and increases epidermal permeability to topically applied agents.

Glycolic acid is the most frequently used AHA for skin care in the United States. It is a natural derivative of sugar cane and contains a single carbon atom. Pharmaceutical preparations of glycolic acid are derived in the laboratory from a reaction between carbon monoxide and formaldehyde. It is produced both as a solution and as a gel. Concentrations of 8% to 14% are formulated for daily skin care. Concentrations of 30% to 70% are used as superficial peeling agents.

Clinically, glycolic preparations are safer than TCA peels, but they must nevertheless be respected. Higher concentrations of glycolic acid can penetrate the dermis. Several cases of hypertrophic scarring following glycolic acid peels have been reported.

Factors affecting the depth of penetration of a glycolic peel include solution concentration, method of application, volume of acid delivered, skin pretreatment, and duration the acid is in contact with the skin. It should be noted that even though 50% solutions are "safer" than 70% solutions, a 50% solution will produce dermal penetration and wounding if left in prolonged contact with the skin. Hence all glycolic acid peels must be vigilantly monitored by the physician and the effects of the acid neutralized when the appropriate depth is reached. In our practice we use water as the neutralizing agent. When the desired depth is reached, the skin is copiously irrigated to arrest the progression of the peel and to remove the acid from the skin's surface. Products with an alkaline pH, usually containing 1% to 15% sodium bicarbonate, may also be used.

Most physicians use 70% solutions of AHAs for chemical peeling agents. Our aesthetician uses 30% solutions for mild peeling; we use 50% solutions for the occasional patient with sensitive skin. Physicians not well versed in the technique of chemical peeling may wish to gain experience with 50% solutions. The gel formulas are the easiest to work with since they can be rapidly applied and do not drip or run onto surfaces not to be treated.

Recognizing the end point of the peel is critical for limiting complications following glycolic peeling. The key is to know the visual stages as they relate to the depth of penetration. An appropriate end point should be selected prior to the application of solution, and the peel should be neutralized when the clinical changes associated with that particular level are visualized. We use these peels as superficial agents and limit their penetration to the epidermis and/or the most superficial level of the papillary dermis. Deeper penetration with glycolic acids is less predictable than with these other modalities and hence there is a narrower margin of safety. Patients showing more severe signs of photoaging should be considered for laser or TCA resurfacing.

As the solution is applied, the skin initially becomes pink and then progressively redder. These changes correspond to epidermal penetration. With time, the epidermal-dermal junction is penetrated; this point is visualized as small areas of gray-white patches. Deeper levels of penetration correspond to true white frosting and signify dermal involvement.

Technique, Postpeel Care, and Complications

The patient's skin is pretreated for 6 to 8 weeks with Retin-A and hydroquinones. The skin is cleansed of dirt and makeup and degreased with alcohol or acetone. We generally use 70% gel solutions applied rapidly to the entire face with well-saturated cotton balls. Since the peel is neutralized with water all at once, it is important to get the chemical in contact with the entire surface as quickly as possible to ensure an even peel. A lag time of even a minute between the first area of application and the last is capable of producing peels of varying depths. We begin by applying the solution to the forehead and rapidly complete the application to the rest of the face. The forehead seems to tolerate the longer contact times the best, and this approach permits shorter contact times on the less forgiving areas of the face.

Safety in glycolic peeling is a function of recognizing the depth of penetration and knowing when to neutralize the acid. Seventy percent solutions left in contact for 5 to 7 minutes on thin, atrophic skin can produce deep peels approaching those seen with medium-depth 35% TCA peels and are best avoided. A patient with thick, sebaceous skin may respond appropriately to 70% solutions left in contact with facial skin for 7 minutes, whereas a patient with thin, dry skin may show similar results with 30% to 50% solutions applied for only 3 to 4 minutes. Patients with superficial pigmentations with few or no rhytides require shorter, lighter peels. Patients with more advanced pathology require (and tolerate) longer contact times and deeper penetration.

The patient will experience mild tingling and stinging during the peel. When the end point is reached, the acid is neutralized using copious cool water irrigation. It is important to use large volumes of water to ensure no residual acid remains on the skin.

Lighter epidermal peels produce only mild flaking and may be covered with a moisturizer and makeup. The use of AHAs or Retin-A is generally discontinued for several days until better tolerated by the freshly treated skin. These peels can be repeated every 1 to 3 weeks as desired. Patients showing early favorable responses are continued on a series of four to six peels or until no additional improvement is obtained. Patients exhibiting little response after the first or second peel should probably be considered for a more aggressive resurfacing modality.

For deeper glycolic peels that produce dermal injury, open petrolatum-based dressings similar to those used after TCA peels are necessary. UV protection should be stressed to avoid hyperpigmentation and maintain the result.

Other regions involved such as the neck, chest, arms, and dorsal surfaces of the hands can be treated with glycolic acids. Pigmentary dyschromias in these regions can be lightened or eliminated with a series of less aggressive treatments. We generally use 30% to 50% solutions and shorter durations for these sites. The end point is signaled by mild erythema and tingling.

Complications from glycolic acid peels generally increase with the depth of the wound. True epidermal wounds consistent with superficial peeling are associated with few complications. Postpeel hyperpigmentation and prolonged erythema are the most common problems, but in our practice they have been rare. Deeper peels extending into the dermis are associated with the same complications seen with other peels of these depths, but again we have rarely experienced this problem.

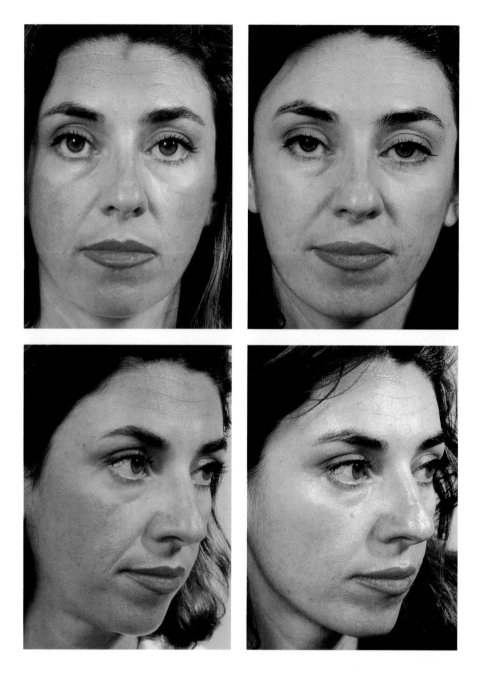

This patient demonstrates some of the typical changes seen following actinic exposure in younger persons. Note the dull, tired appearance of the skin surface associated with blotchy pigmentary irregularities. She is shown following three 70% glycolic acid peels at 2-week intervals. A comprehensive skin care program, ultraviolet avoidance, sunscreens, 4% hydroquinone, and Retin-A supplemented the glycolic peels. Note the improvement in pigmentary irregularities, a brighter, fresher skin appearance, and diminution of the fine rhytides.

MicroPeel

The MicroPeel by BioMedic combines mechanical removal of the outer keratin layers of the epidermis with superficial chemical exfoliation using AHA. The MicroPeel program consists of a series of treatments generally performed at 2-week intervals. It is useful for ameliorating mild pigmentary irregularities and freshening the skin's appearance and texture. We also use this system as an adjunct to skin preparation prior to deeper TCA or laser resurfacing. This procedure may be performed by a trained aesthetician. The skin is thoroughly cleansed, and the outer layer of keratin is mechanically removed with a Bio-Medic dermaplaning blade while the skin is held under tension. The outer keratinized layer of skin is "dermaplaned" away as thin sheets of skin rolling off the edge of the blade.

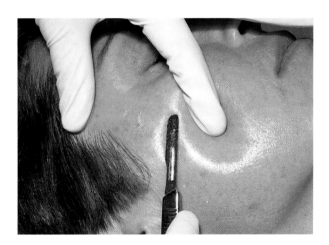

The patient's skin is held under tension between the thumb and index finger of the physician's nondominant hand while the dermaplane blade is moved tangentially across the skin surface. Sheets of dead outer keratin are mechanically removed, allowing the glycolic acid to penetrate to deeper depths.

Women should be informed beforehand that this process will remove facial hair in the dermaplaned areas. Some patients will find this objectionable. In men the MicroPeel process is performed over a freshly shaved beard.

A 30% solution of glycolic acid is applied to the skin's surface following mechanical removal of the keratin layer. Similar parameters to those discussed for routine glycolic acid peels are used to judge time and depth, but as a rule, peels performed by the aesthetician with 30% solutions are limited to a few minutes for a greater margin of safety. When the peel is terminated, dry ice is lightly brushed over the face for a soothing effect and to aid in neutralization of the acid. The procedure is completed with the application of a moisturizer that contains a sunscreen. Patients may return immediately to their normal routine with only mild flaking or redness.

Trichloroacetic Acid

TCA in concentrations of 10% to 20% is classified as a light peeling agent. Light TCA peels may be performed in patients who have mild actinic changes and in those who cannot afford a longer recovery time. In addition to the traditional facial peeling, concentrations in this range make TCA suitable for use in actinically damaged regions of the neck and anterior chest.

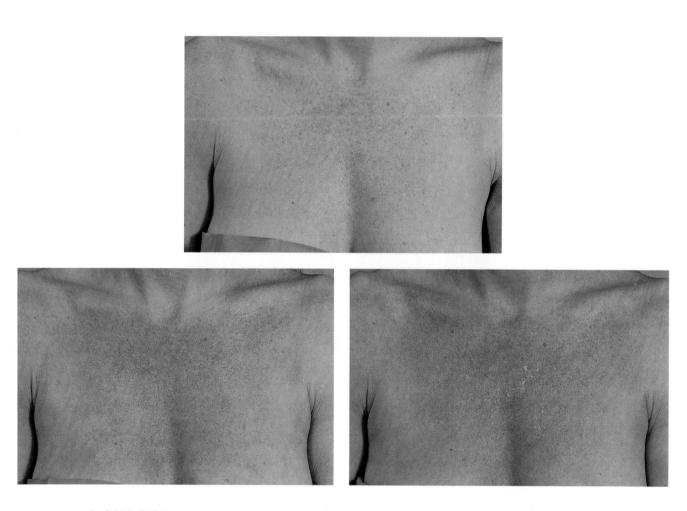

A 20% TCA concentration was used to treat early actinic changes in this patient's presternal skin. Generalized erythema without frosting is evident 90 seconds following a single TCA application. At 3 minutes spotty frosting and intensification of the background erythema can be observed, representing the clinical end point of superficial peeling on the anterior chest wall.

TCA in any concentration is capable of producing wounds well into the dermis. Experience and judgment are necessary to recognize the clinical signs indicating peel depth and selection of patients based on skin thickness and anticipated response to the peeling agent. As the concentration of the acid is increased, the rate of wounding is likewise increased. Similarly, as additional coats of acid are applied, the depth of wounding is increased. When used as a superficial peeling agent, a single light application is usually all that is required.

The indications for superficial peeling using 10% to 20% TCA are similar to those conditions responding to glycolic acid peels. To achieve the desired clinical effect, superficial TCA peels will need to be repeated at frequent intervals. Pretreatment with Retin-A will enhance the effectiveness of superficial TCA peels. (See Chapter 5 for more detailed information on TCA.)

Salicylic Acid

Salicylic acid peels are less popular than the other available agents because they are cumbersome and require more labor-intensive care. Salicylic acid is available as a 50% paste for peeling the arms and hands. It is used in Jessner's solution at 14% strength. Only one upper extremity is peeled at any session to avoid toxicity and the development of salicylism. The skin is vigorously cleansed with acetone, and raised keratoses are treated individually with 20% TCA spot peeling. The volar surfaces of the forearm and the web spaces of the fingers are protected with occlusive tape. The 50% paste is applied to the exposed dorsal surfaces of the forearm and hand. The paste is occluded with plastic wrap and then covered with Kerlix or an Ace wrap and left in place for 48 hours. Patients should be given a checklist to alert them to signs and symptoms of salicylism. The bandages are removed at 48 hours and the excess paste removed. The arms and hands are covered with antibiotic ointment and gauze. This process is repeated until the wounds heal in 7 to 14 days.

ROLE OF THE AESTHETICIAN

Incorporating an aesthetician into an aesthetic surgery practice can improve the quality of skin care that the patient receives and increase the consistency of results after deep resurfacing. This professional plays a valuable role during the entire treatment process, helping to evaluate, educate, and treat the patient while monitoring and promoting compliance and a smooth postoperative course.

Patients who seek treatment for photodamaged skin are seen in consultation with the aesthetician, who evaluates the dermal pathology and familiarizes the patient with products available for daily skin care. If TCA peeling or deep resurfacing is contemplated, the aesthetician assists in formulating the pretreatment regimen appropriate for the individual patient's skin type and lifestyle.

Sufficient time is allowed for the aesthetician to properly educate patients and instruct them in product use. The aesthetician will also usually see a patient several times prior to peeling or resurfacing to ensure that the skin care program is being carried out properly.

Our aesthetician performs superficial peels, including MicroPeels (mechanical abrasion), Jessner's peels, 30% glycolic peels, and 10% TCA peels. For these types of superficial peels, patients are scheduled at 2- to 3-week intervals. She also instructs the patient in daily skin care to maintain the results.

After deep resurfacing and surgical rejuvenation, the aesthetician consults with the patient on the use of camouflaging makeup. Makeup can usually be applied 10 days after treatment and permits the patient to resume normal daily activities. Instructing the patient about makeup, use of sunscreens, and resumption of a posttreatment Retin-A and hydroquinone program is critical to the prevention of hyperpigmentation.

Few procedures in plastic surgery are as labor intensive as skin resurfacing. Patients are evaluated frequently to address their questions and attend to minor problems. The aesthetician is a key staff member for follow-up and alleviating patient concerns. In essence the aesthetician serves as the liaison between physician and patient, identifying problems before they become serious and facilitating patient compliance. Since we have incorporated an aesthetician in our practice our results have improved and patient satisfaction has increased.

CONCLUDING THOUGHTS

Not all skin problems require treatment with middermal resurfacing techniques, nor will all patients accept these more aggressive treatment modalities. Superficial peeling agents are ideal for patients who desire dermatologic improvement with minimal posttreatment morbidity. Although lasting improvement of facial wrinkling is rarely seen following superficial resurfacing, long-term improvement of disorders of facial pigmentation can be obtained. The physician treating sun-damaged skin should be well versed in the plethora of agents available for skin care and superficial peeling in order to most effectively address the needs of each individual patient.

REFERENCES

Autier P, Dore J, Schifflers E, et al. Melanoma and use of sunscreens: An EORTIC case-control study in Germany, Belgium, and France. Int J Cancer 61:749, 1995.

Bark JP. A systematic approach to Retin-A. Facial Plast Surg Clin North Am 2(1):11, 1994.

Brody HJ. Chemical Peeling. St. Louis: Mosby—Year Book, 1992.

Clark CP III, Rohrich RJ. Skin care in an aesthetic plastic surgery practice: Indications and scientific rationale. Perspect Plast Surg 8(1):159, 1994.

Coven RM, Pinnell SR. Topical vitamin C in aging. Clin Dermatol 14:227, 1996.

Darr D, Combs S, Dunston S, et al. Topical vitamin C protects porcine skin from ultraviolet radiation-induced damage. Br J Dermatol 127:247, 1992.

Ellis DAF, Trimas SJ, Ellis CS. The use of glycolic acid as a micro-peel. Facial Plast Surg Clin North Am 2(1):15, 1994.

Gilchrest BA. Skin and Aging Processes. Boca Raton: CRC Press, 1984.

Gregory RO. Coherent UltraPulse Aesthetic Laser Surgery Resurfacing Course. Palo Alto: Coherent, 1995.

Hevia O, Nemeth AJ, Taylor JR. Tretinoin accelerates healing after trichloroacetic acid chemical peel. Arch Dermatol 127:678, 1991.

Kligman AM. Results of a pilot study evaluating the compatibility of topical tretinoin in combination with glycolic acid. Cosmet Dermatol 6(10):28-32, 1993.

Kligman AM, Kligman LH. The treatment of photoaged skin with topical retinoic acid. Perspect Plast Surg 2(2):63, 1988.

Kligman AM, Grove GL, Hirose R, et al. Topical tretinoin for photoaged skin. J Am Acad Dermatol 15:836, 1986.

Monheit GD. The Jessner's-TCA peel. An enhanced medium-depth chemical peel. Facial Plast Surg Clin North Am 2(1):21, 1994.

Monheit GD. Advances in chemical peeling. Facial Plast Surg Clin North Am 2(1):5, 1994.

Montagna W, Kirchner S, Carlisle K. Histology of sun-damaged human skin. J Am Acad Dermatol 21:907, 1989.

Rubin MG. Manual of Chemical Peels: Superficial and Medium Depth. Philadelphia: JB Lippincott, 1992.

Stagnone JJ. Superficial peeling. J Dermatol Surg Oncol 15:924, 1989.

Stuzin JM, Baker TJ, Gordon HL. Treatment of photoaging: Facial chemical peeling (phenol and trichloroacetic acid) and dermabrasion. Clin Plast Surg 20:9, 1993.

Tamima S, Pinnell SR. Ascorbic acid preferentially enhances type I and III collagen gene transcription in human skin fibroblasts. J Dermatol Sci 11:250, 1996.

Topical vitamin C diminishes wrinkles, signs of photoaging. Geriatrics 50(11):23, 1995.

Van Scott EJ, Ruey JY. Hyperkeratinization, corneocyte cohesion, and alpha hydroxy acids. J Am Acad Dermatol 11:867, 1984.

Van Scott EJ, Ruey JY. Alpha hydroxy acids: Procedures for use in clinical practice. Cutis 43:222, 1989.

Weiss JS, Ellis CN, Headington JT, et al. Topical tretinoin improves photoaged skin: A double-blind vehicle-controlled study. JAMA 4:527, 1988.

Weiss JS, Ellis CN, Goldfarb MT, et al. Tretinoin treatment of photodamaged skin: Cosmesis through medical therapy. Dermatol Clin 9:123, 1991.

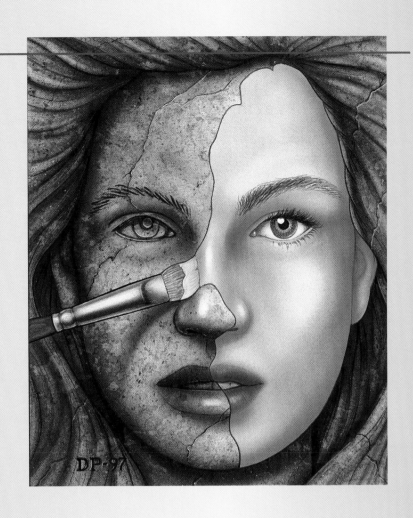

TCA Peels

Perhaps no peeling agent affords the plastic surgeon such versatility and flexibility as trichloroacetic acid (TCA). The unique properties of this agent enable the physician to treat a wide range of patients by varying the depth of each chemical peel. Unlike phenol, TCA appears to have less effect on melanocyte metabolism and thus a decreased tendency for bleaching facial skin. Therefore it can be used for patients with different complexions ranging from those with pale, white Nordic skin to more brunette, Hispanic complexions and also for individuals of East Asian and African origin. The ability to offer dermatologic treatment to patients of various ethnic backgrounds is of great advantage, particularly for physicians who practice in areas with diverse ethnic populations. The minimal morbidity associated with medium-depth TCA peeling with its rapid, painless recovery, lack of systemic absorption, and decreased tendency for bleaching of facial skin makes TCA an appealing alternative for patients who want predictable improvement with minimal disruption of their daily routines.

As plastic surgeons have become increasingly aware of the benefits of the TCA peels that their dermatologic colleagues have long favored, TCA peels have begun to supplant the traditional phenol peels. At the current time we perform a much larger number of TCA peels than we do phenol peels, which represents a significant change in our practice pattern. Although in our long experience with phenol peeling we demonstrated largely reliable and predictable responses, the prolonged perioperative morbidity and postpeel erythema could not be ignored. The high degree of patient satisfaction associated with medium-depth TCA peeling and the rapid recovery have prompted us to use this agent with greater frequency.

TCA peels range from superficial to deep depending on the concentration used. Superficial peeling agents in 10% to 20% concentrations are primarily exfoliants affecting the outer layers of the epidermis. Medium-depth peels in concentrations ranging from 30% to 40% penetrate the papillary dermis and are the most commonly used because they offer the advantages of low morbidity and predictable recovery. These peels are useful for treating a broad spectrum of problems ranging from pigmentation disorders to fine facial rhytides. Deep TCA peels in concentrations ranging from 40% to 50% solution penetrate the reticular dermis and are used to treat coarse facial rhytides and pigmentation disorders localized to the deep portion of the dermis. These peels are associated with greater morbidity and a longer recovery period.

TCA peels have their limitations. In patients with coarse facial rhytides, especially in the perioral region, we have found the results of TCA peeling to be disappointing. Also, unlike phenol peeling or laser resurfacing, the long-term effects of TCA peels may be more transitory; many patients will demonstrate initial improvement only to require additional peeling after several months.

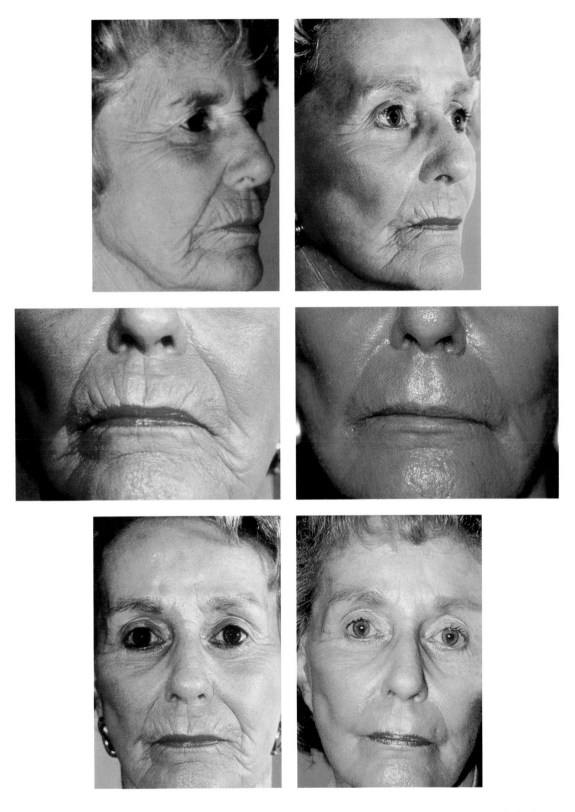

This patient is seen before and after a 35% medium-depth TCA peel with little improvement in the perioral region. Subsequently, we performed another medium-depth peel combined with a perioral phenol peel. The final result shows the improvement that can be obtained using a combination of treatment modalities.

In contrast to phenol peeling, there is a significant learning curve associated with mastering the TCA technique. Phenol produces an all-or-none response and a prepeel preparation is not required. A single application of the Baker-Gordon phenol formula to unprepared skin produces uniform dermal penetration associated with predictable neocollagen formation. Consistent results can be expected as long as the correct phenol formula has been used. The greatest limitation of phenol peeling is that it is not applicable for an ethnically diverse patient population. TCA, on the other hand, demands more technical skill and clinical judgment. Penetration is affected by the concentration of the solution, prepeel preparation of facial skin, perioperative degreasing, the number of coats of peeling agent applied, and the method of application. Only through experience can the depth of TCA penetration be judged. The ability to "read the peel" is key to mastering this technique and ensuring safe and predictable results.

INDICATIONS

TCA peels can be used to treat a wide variety of dermatologic conditions. We have found them to be particularly suited for patients with pigmentation disorders and actinically damaged skin. We have also used TCA for diffuse epidermal dysplasias of the face and for acne scarring as an adjunctive treatment to dermabrasion.

Pigmentation Disorders

Blotchy facial skin is the common denominator that characterizes a wide variety of clinical problems classified as facial pigmentation disorders. Injuries of many types can produce disorders of facial pigmentation, including chronic actinic damage, the hormonal changes produced by pregnancy or birth control pills, viral exanthems, or chronic inflammatory conditions such as acne scarring. Patients with these problems tend to be classified as having Fitzpatrick types III to IV skin; they respond to ultraviolet insult by tanning rather than burning. These patients have a substantial number of melanocytes within the epidermis and tend to form pigment in response to injury. If the pigment is laid down unevenly, the facial skin becomes blotchy.

Disorders of facial skin pigmentation will respond to a number of different peeling agents provided that most of the melanocytic pigment is within the range of the peel depth. If blotchy pigmentation is secondary to melanocytic deposition localized to the basal layer of the epidermis, then superficial and medium-depth peeling agents can effectively treat this problem. Some disorders of pigmentation, however, will be accompanied by the presence of reticular dermal pigment, and while improving these conditions, superficial or medium-depth peeling will leave residual pigmentation. For this reason, it is important for the physician to understand the depth of pigmentation prior to selecting the appropriate peeling agent.

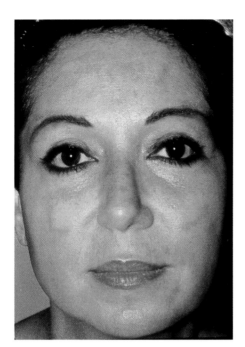 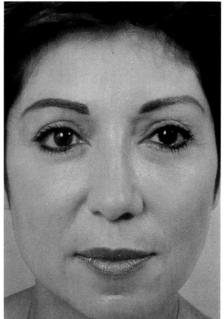

This patient exhibits splotchy hyperpigmentation secondary to chronic sun exposure. Because of her basically dark complexion and the likelihood of postpeel hyperpigmentation, prolonged pretreatment with Retin-A and hydroquinone was required. The postpeel result is seen following a single 35% TCA peel taken to a medium depth. The facial improvement has been maintained over the past several years without the need for a repeat TCA peel. A daily skin care program and sun avoidance have contributed to the longevity of the result.

We have found it useful to fluoresce the skin with Wood's light to evaluate patients with pigmentation disorders. Wood's light allows the clinician to accurately assess the depth and location of the pathology. If the pigmentation is localized to the epidermis, a skin care routine and superficial peeling are often successful. Pigmentation problems that involve the papillary dermis often can be treated with medium-depth TCA peeling.

Pretreatment with agents that suppress melanocytic metabolism is key when using TCA to treat disorders of hyperpigmentation. Patients with disorders of pigmentation tend to respond to any form of dermal injury by forming pigment. This response must be suppressed prior to stimulating dermal healing via any form of resurfacing. TCA peeling can either improve or produce blotchy hyperpigmentation depending on how the individual responds to the insult of TCA application. Pretreatment using a combination of Retin-A and hydroquinone to promote uniform pigmentation on healing is requisite to consistent results.

Photoaged Skin and Rhytides

Photoaging refers to the histologic and cosmetic changes resulting from repeated sun exposure rather than those associated with the passage of time. The photoaged epidermis is characterized by atrophy; the stratum corneum is thickened and the epithelium becomes dysplastic secondary to chronic ultraviolet injury. Melanocytic hypertrophy is a common histologic finding that makes actinically damaged skin appear blotchy and is responsible for the presence of solar lentigines or age spots. Actinic damage of the dermis causes collagen degeneration as well as degeneration of dermal elastic fibers. Clinically, the skin has a leathery texture and exhibits coarse and fine wrinkling.

The epidermal effects of photoaging will commonly respond to a single medium-depth TCA peel or can be treated by multiple superficial peels performed at frequent intervals. We prefer medium-depth peeling for treating facial pigmentation problems because the results of a single treatment are usually predictable. For other chronically actinically damaged areas such as the chest, back, neck, or extremities, in which the adnexal structures for healing are not as numerous, we prefer to treat the epidermal types of actinic injuries by performing frequent superficial TCA peels. These types of peels, usually performed with 20% to 30% TCA solutions, are taken to the level of the basement layer of the epidermis. They are associated with minimal morbidity and can safely be repeated at biweekly intervals.

The dermal signs of sun damage are manifest clinically as facial rhytides. Medium-depth TCA peeling appears to be a predictable treatment for fine facial rhytides. The results of peeling in patients with coarse facial rhytides are less reliable. If TCA is used to treat coarse rhytides, the peeling agent must penetrate deep to the papillary dermis, and reticular dermal peels are associated with greater patient morbidity. In our experience the neocollagen formation following upper reticular dermal TCA peeling is less predictable than that obtained with phenol or laser resurfacing; the response of coarse facial rhytides to TCA peeling is inconsistent, especially in the perioral region. When treating rhytides within the cheeks, periorbital region, and forehead, however, we have achieved a more predictable response with upper reticular dermal TCA peels. Individualization of treatment planning and use of a combination of modalities will produce more consistent results.

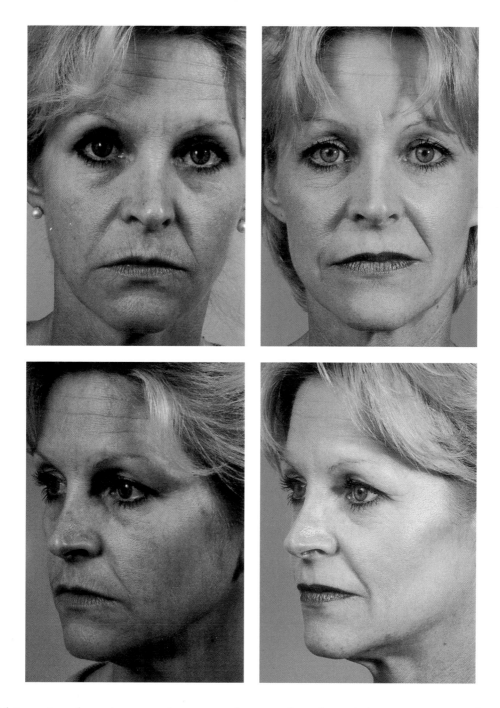

This patient has pigmentation secondary to chronic actinic exposure associated with rhytides of the upper lip. A combination of treatment modalities were used, including prepeel preparation with Retin-A and hydroquinone, two medium-depth 35% TCA peels, dermabrasion of the upper lip, and a maintenance skin program of Retin-A, glycolic acid creams, and sunscreens. She is shown 15 months following the initial treatment.

The results of TCA treatment of facial rhytides are not as long lasting as with phenol treatment. Although many patients will exhibit an excellent response in the immediate postpeel period, residual rhytides will be noticeable at 6-month to 1-year follow-up. The more transient nature of the TCA results may be attributable to less neocollagen formation after peeling as well as its effect on epidermal and dermal hydration. Initially TCA peeling seems to restore normal dermal hydration, and the postpeel edema acts to conceal the appearance of fine facial wrinkling. Over time, however, the dermal hydration stimulated by the TCA peel diminishes and facial wrinkles may reappear. Reapplication of medium-depth TCA peeling solution often restores the improved clinical appearance of these patients.

Epidermal Dysplasias

Disorders of epidermal proliferation, loss of epidermal vertical cell polarity, development of actinic keratoses, and preinvasive basal cell carcinoma are all examples of epidermal changes secondary to actinic damage. Any treatment modality that totally removes the epidermis to permit regeneration of a more normal-appearing epidermis will improve the appearance of patients with these disorders. TCA, phenol, laser resurfacing, and dermabrasion all produce an injury deep to the basement layer of the epidermis; for this reason, all four agents can be used to treat epidermal dysplasias.

Epidermal dysplasias are commonly treated with fluorouracil rather than chemical peeling. However, peeling may be appropriate for the occasional patient with severe actinic damage associated with multiple actinic keratoses affecting the entire face. In these individuals TCA peeling taken at least to the papillary dermis will ameliorate multiple actinic keratoses and improve the appearance of the actinically damaged skin. Careful follow-up of these individuals is crucial since these peels can be repeated at regular intervals as clinically warranted. We find medium-depth peeling preferable to surgical resection or fluorouracil in patients with a large number of actinic keratoses since there seems to be less morbidity associated with a medium-depth peel than other forms of treatment. Medium-depth peeling with TCA is not appropriate for basal cell carcinoma, and patients who are prone to form cancers must be followed systematically if this modality is chosen.

Acne Scarring

Acne scarring represents a cluster of clinical problems for which there is no ideal treatment. Patients usually have thick, sebaceous skin that is firm and fibrotic from chronic inflammatory changes. In our experience most patients will respond in varying degrees to a series of dermabrasion or laser treatments for ameliorating the appearance of their pockmarks. If patients have previously had dermabrasion, reticular dermal peels with TCA will provide some improvement of residual scars. To obtain consistent dermal peels in these patients requires an excellent pretreatment regimen. These peels should be performed with the patient under sedation using concentrations of 35% to 45% TCA solution.

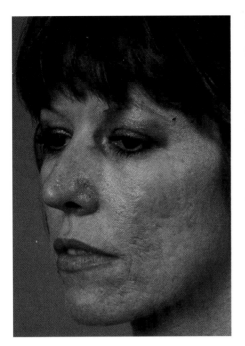 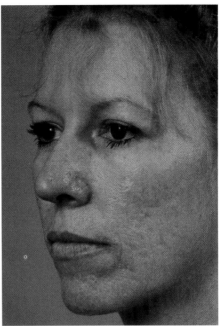

This patient exemplifies the use of TCA peeling to treat acne scars. Typically, following TCA peeling patients with acne scarring will exhibit an overall improvement in the texture of their skin, and commonly the postinflammatory pigmentation associated with this condition will improve. Although dermabrasion or laser resurfacing is perhaps a better treatment modality for deep pockmarks in our opinion, the decreased morbidity of TCA peeling makes it suitable for treating patients with more limited and shallow scars.

EVALUATION OF SKIN TYPE

The planning and outcome of TCA peeling must take into consideration skin thickness and texture and facial pigmentation. Evaluation of these factors is essential for planning the best approach for TCA peeling.

Skin Thickness and Texture

Skin thickness and texture will influence how rapidly the peel penetrates the skin. Patients with thick, oily skin tolerate the TCA application better; in these patients higher concentrations of TCA or multiple reapplications of the chemical agent will be necessary to obtain the appropriate level of peel penetration. In patients with oily skin prepeel degreasing is especially important for ensuring uniform penetration.

Conversely, TCA penetration can occur rapidly in patients with thin, dry skin that appears atrophic and fragile in texture. In such patients this factor must be taken into account to prevent wounding into the deep dermis, particularly if the patient has been properly pretreated with prolonged use of Retin-A. Hypertrophic scarring is most common in these types of patients because of failure to control the rapid penetration of the peeling agent beyond the desired level of impact.

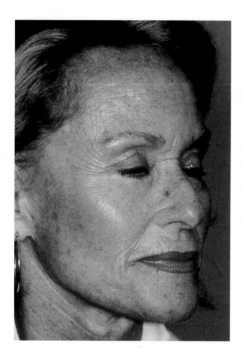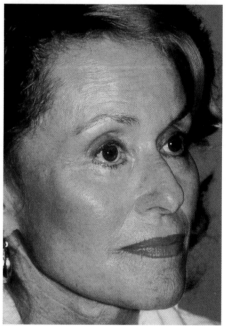

Skin thickness and texture influence the depth of penetration of TCA. This patient has splotchy hyperpigmentation and fine facial wrinkling secondary to chronic actinic exposure. Her skin is thin and dry. She was placed on a standard prepeel regimen before peeling with a single 35% TCA application. Care was taken to avoid deep dermal penetration beyond the level desired. Medium-depth peeling has led to a predictable improvement of the splotchy pigmentation.

Facial Pigmentation

The most common sequelae of TCA peeling is postinflammatory hyperpigmentation. Certain types of patients are more at risk for this troublesome problem, and evaluation of skin type will help prevent this complication. Patients with Fitzpatrick types I and II skin (white in color and with a tendency to burn rather than tan in response to actinic exposure) are not prone to postpeel hyperpigmentation, even if not properly pretreated with Retin-A and hydroquinone.

The potential for postpeel hyperpigmentation becomes more likely when treating patients with a darker complexion. This is especially true in olive-skinned, brown-eyed individuals who tan easily but do not burn in response to ultraviolet light and in patients of East Asian or African descent. Patients with disorders of pigmentation such as melasma are at risk of developing postpeel hyperpigmentation if epidermal melanocytes are not suppressed prior to peeling.

It is important to place patients with darker complexions or those with facial pigmentation disorders on a skin care program to suppress melanocytes prior to resurfacing. Patients, however, are not always compliant. For this reason, it is appropriate to schedule several appointments to see the patient prior to peeling to ensure that the pretreatment regimen is followed. Use of a staff aesthetician is helpful for monitoring the patient. We sometimes treat these patients initially with superficial peels to check their response prior to performing deeper peels. If the results achieved with epidermal and papillary dermal peels are good and the patient does not develop hyperpigmentation, a deeper peel can be performed if needed at a later date.

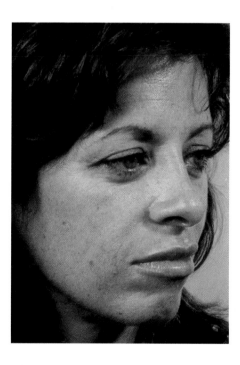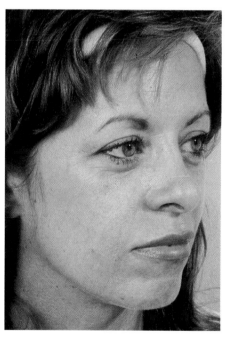

Patients with splotchy hyperpigmentation localized to the epidermis and superficial dermis respond favorably to TCA peels. This patient is shown following a single medium-depth 35% TCA peel after appropriate prepeel skin preparation. Postpeel skin care, sunscreens, and sun avoidance are essential to maintain the results.

PREPEEL REGIMEN

Consistent results with TCA peeling depend on prepeel preparation. TCA is a milder peeling agent than phenol and shows less consistent penetration of the epidermal-dermal junction. Pretreatment of facial skin improves the ability of TCA to penetrate beyond the protective stratum corneum of the epidermis and deep to the epidermal-dermal junction.

Pretreatment enhances the uniform uptake of the peeling solution, leading to uniform healing and consistent results. Prepeel treatment is also essential to suppress melanocyte metabolism and prevent postpeel hyperpigmentation. Retin-A is the cornerstone of our prepeel treatment regimen. It has profound effects on epidermal metabolism, causing increased cellular proliferation, suppression of melanocyte hyperactivity, and thinning of the stratum corneum. The changes produced by Retin-A result in more rapid and uniform penetration of the TCA and more rapid healing following the peel by enhancing cellular proliferation.

In patients with Fitzpatrick types III to V skin we strongly recommend adding hydroquinone to the prepeel regimen. Hydroquinone affects melanocytic metabolism by decreasing melanin formation and increasing the degradation of melanocyte pigment; it inhibits tyrosinase, the hormone responsible for increasing the proliferation of melanocytes. Depigmentation does not occur immediately following hydroquinone application because this chemical interferes only with the formation of new melanin. The effectiveness of hydroquinone is enhanced by the simultaneous use of Retin-A, which appears to increase the penetration of the hydroquinone and works synergistically to suppress melanocytic metabolism. Pretreating patients with both of these chemical agents enhances uniform pigmentation following peeling and helps prevent postpeel hyperpigmentation.

Retin-A Cream

The initial pretreatment plan begins with applications of 0.1% Retin-A. Because of the potential irritant effects associated with Retin-A and possible problems with patient compliance should retinoid dermatitis develop, we first prescribe a small amount of this cream and then gradually increase the frequency and volume of application as tolerated. We instruct patients to apply a small amount of cream to the entire face at bedtime (usually a volume comparable to a pea or small grape). Most can tolerate this concentration of Retin-A every other night. Patients tend not to apply the Retin-A uniformly to the face but rather concentrate on those areas of their complexion that they find most troubling, such as areas of facial wrinkling. Obviously spotty application of Retin-A will result in spotty uptake of the peeling solution. Therefore we stress uniform application over the face, including the lower lid and crow's-feet area, reaching up to the hairline and extending into the preauricular area of the cheeks. If the neck or chest is to be peeled, additional Retin-A should be applied to these areas (see Chapter 4).

Hydroquinone Cream

If postinflammatory pigmentation is a concern, we add nightly applications of 4% hydroquinone cream to the regimen. Hydroquinone, similar to Retin-A, is applied uniformly over the face in the same volume. We usually have the patient mix an equal volume of Retin-A and hydroquinone together and apply this mixture evenly over the entire facial surface. In patients who have disorders of hyperpigmentation or who have a dark complexion, the hydroquinone is used twice daily, both at night with the Retin-A and in the morning as a solitary agent before applying a sunscreen.

Sunscreens

The use of sunscreens is imperative in all patients undergoing prepeel treatment. Retin-A sensitizes the skin to sun exposure and makes the patient more vulnerable to actinic damage if the skin is not adequately protected. In patients who are undergoing peeling for hyperpigmentation the sunscreens work synergistically with hydroquinone and Retin-A to protect against ultraviolet (UV)-induced melanocytic hypertrophy. We recommend using sunscreens that block not only UVB light but also UVA light (Shade-UVA).

Duration of Pretreatment Regimen

The duration of the pretreatment regimen varies from patient to patient. Since epidermal cell cycles are approximately 45 days, we believe the pretreatment program should be continued for at least 6 weeks so that the topical creams have a maximal effect on the newly formed cells. If deep reticular dermal peels are planned, we prefer to pretreat for at least two cell cycles, that is, at least 3 months prior to TCA application.

Alternate Treatment Regimen

The alpha hydroxy acids (AHAs) are naturally occurring acids found in many foods. When patients cannot tolerate Retin-A, we often substitute glycolic acid, an AHA derived from sugar cane. We start them on twice-daily applications of glycolic acid solution usually ranging from 10% to 14% in concentration. If the patient tolerates the glycolic applications, we add hydroquinone creams to the routine; these are usually applied nightly but can be used twice a day in patients with hyperpigmentation. Although we prefer Retin-A over glycolic acid for pretreatment prior to TCA peeling, we are satisfied with the effect of glycolic acid, especially in patients in whom only papillary dermal peeling is planned as opposed to deep reticular dermal peels. Glycolic acid acts primarily to thin the stratum corneum and enhance uniform TCA penetration. When used in conjunction with hydroquinone, melanocytic suppression is enhanced, similar to combined Retin-A/hydroquinone pretreatment.

CHOICE OF AGENTS

One of the distinct advantages of TCA peels is that the depth of peeling can be varied according to the specific needs and wishes of the patient. In active patients who desire minimal recovery and are only seeking a fresher skin appearance, superficial peeling is appropriate. In these individuals a 20% single application of TCA, with or without pretreatment, is often satisfactory. These patients can have these "freshening" peels done at frequent intervals if desired. Although little risk is associated with superficial peels, the results are often limited.

In patients with pigmentation problems confined to the epidermis and superficial dermis, medium-depth peeling is appropriate. Patients with actinically damaged skin and fine facial rhytides will have a good response to medium-depth peels to the level of the papillary dermis. Consistent results can usually be obtained in these patients if a proper pretreatment skin program is followed and a 35% TCA solution is used for peeling.

In patients with severe actinic damage and coarse facial rhytides, significant epidermal dysplasia, thick, oily skin, or acne-type scarring, deeper (upper reticular dermal) peels are appropriate. We usually perform these deeper peels with the patient sedated. We typically use a modified 40% to 45% TCA solution. On occasion we have used a 50% TCA solution but find that this concentration is difficult to control because of its potential for rapid penetration into the dermis. Rapid penetration also impedes the ability to "read the peel" and accurately judge the depth of penetration of the peeling agent. For this reason, we use a modified 50% TCA solution formulated as follows:

> *Modified TCA Solution*
> 5 ml of 50% TCA
> 1 ml glycerin
> 8 drops Tween 20

This modified solution produces a concentration of TCA in the 40% to 45% range. The glycerin helps ensure a smooth, uniform application of the peeling agent, and the Tween 20 acts as a surfactant to keep the TCA and glycerin in solution. The addition of the glycerin delays TCA penetration so that the physician is able to accurately judge the depth of penetration of the peeling agent and determine if another application of solution is appropriate.

TCA solutions will vary depending on the pharmacy supplying it; therefore a 35% solution from one pharmacy may act differently from a 35% solution from another. We would suggest that physicians just beginning to perform TCA peels seek a pharmacist who has experience in preparing TCA solutions or order specific TCA concentrations from a national pharmacy distributor. In our office we keep a variety of TCA strengths available, ranging from 20% to 50% concentrations.

The importance of knowing the exact concentration of the TCA solution used cannot be overemphasized. We have had several patients referred to us for hypertrophic scarring whose physicians claim that only a 35% concentration was used. Although many factors affect the penetration of TCA, we suspect that the pharmacist may not have accurately prepared the TCA mixture. If the physician does not have a reliable and dependable pharmacist that he has worked with, it is advisable that TCA be obtained through a national distributor.

TECHNIQUE
Skin Preparation and Degreasing

The skin must be properly prepared before the application of any peeling agent. The patient is instructed to arrive at the office without makeup or to remove any residual makeup. The skin is then carefully cleansed with an acetone-containing solution to remove residual oils; this is usually followed by wiping with an alcohol sponge prior to peel application. In patients with thick, oily skin or in those who require a deeper peel, we find it helpful to mechanically abrade the skin gently with a gauze sponge soaked in acetone. This mechanical abrasion removes the stratum corneum, thereby contributing to a more uniform penetration of the peeling agent.

SUPERFICIAL PEELS

Epidermal peels are performed using a 20% TCA solution. Although pretreatment with Retin-A is preferable, it is not obligatory. A single application of 20% solution uniformly applied to the face will produce erythema or mild frosting. Following application the patient can wash her face to dilute the peeling agent and then apply a light moisturizer if required. The patient's face will usually exhibit mild flaking or desquamation for 3 to 5 days as well as postpeel erythema for a similar time interval. There are no limitations on activity during this period and patients may wear makeup. These types of peels are accurately called "refresher" peels. However, if they are performed at frequent intervals in conjunction with the daily use of Retin-A, glycolic acid, and hydroquinone, clinical improvement of actinically damaged skin will be noted.

Superficial peels are described in more detail in Chapter 4.

MEDIUM-DEPTH PEELS

TCA in various concentrations can be used to penetrate the basement layer of the epidermis and produce dermal peeling. We carry these so-called medium-depth peels to the level of the papillary dermis, although they can extend to the uppermost portion of the reticular dermis. If the skin is properly prepared with topical creams and these peels are performed in a regional fashion, sedation is usually unnecessary.

We generally use a 35% TCA solution for these types of peels. A moderately soaked 2 × 2 inch gauze sponge is used to apply the peeling solution in a series of crosshatching strokes using firm, even pressure. When the patient is not sedated, the solution is applied regionally—forehead, right cheek, left cheek, perioral region, and nose—to each facial unit. Most patients are able to tolerate 1 to 2 minutes of discomfort if the pain is localized to a specific region. Fanning the patient vigorously as the peeling solution is applied helps alleviate the burning sensation as the peel is applied. The patient can be premedicated with extra-strength Tylenol or Darvocet if required. If the skin has been properly prepared with Retin-A, adequate penetration of the peeling solution usually occurs within 60 to 120 seconds. Once the desired degree of frosting and penetration is obtained, the peel is lavaged with ice water to increase patient comfort.

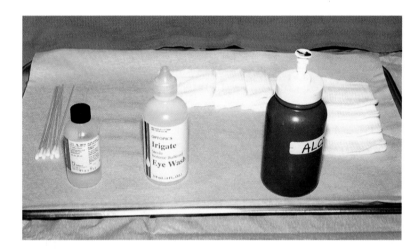

A peel tray is assembled before beginning medium-depth TCA peeling. The face is degreased meticulously with either alcohol or acetone. The peel solution is applied with both gauze and sponges, and Q-tips are available to apply the solution to areas such as the lower eyelid. Eyewash solution is always kept on this tray should ophthalmic lavage be required.

"Reading the Peel"

The key to safe and consistent TCA peels is adequately judging the depth of penetration of the peeling solution. Three clinical signs assist in determining the depth of penetration: (1) degree of frosting, (2) skin turgor, and (3) return of skin color following resolution of frosting. There is a definite learning curve involved in TCA peeling. The physician's understanding of these three factors will control the depth of penetration of the TCA, thereby producing the desired effect.

Frosting

The skin's appearance after the peeling solution is applied is perhaps the key element in judging depth of penetration and ability to read the peel. When TCA is applied in light concentrations (20%), it produces an erythematous reaction. As the peeling solution penetrates to the basement layer of the epidermis, a uniform pink/white frosting occurs. Penetration deep to the basement membrane is associated with a deeper white frost that is characteristic of penetration into the papillary dermis. Penetration deep to the papillary dermis associated with reticular dermal peels produces a uniformly dense, opaque white frost. If the peel penetrates deeper in the reticular dermis, the skin assumes a gray appearance, which is a danger sign signaling deep dermal penetration and the potential for healing with hypertrophic scarring.

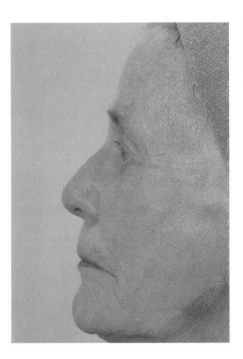 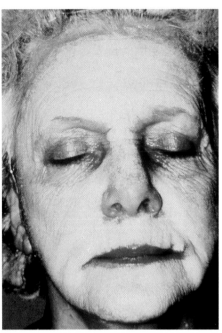

The degree of frosting is the prime indicator of the depth of penetration. The patient on the left is shown following a 30% TCA peel taken to the level of the junction between epidermis and papillary dermis. Note the uniform pink/white frosting that is fairly light in color. The patient on the right exhibits the dense white frosting seen after TCA penetration into the papillary dermis.

There is a time lag between peel application and the maximum degree of frosting that occurs following a single application of TCA. This time interval will vary from patient to patient but is approximately 45 to 90 seconds. For this reason, when performing medium to deep TCA peels, it is important to wait at least 45 seconds to judge the depth of frosting before applying another coat of TCA solution. *Judging the degree of frosting requires patience but is perhaps the single best guide in preventing unwanted deep penetration of the peeling agent.*

Skin Turgor

As the peel solution penetrates facial skin, the skin develops a different turgor or feel on palpation. Untreated skin is soft and mobile to the touch. In light peels the skin turgor increases, and the smooth, sliding facial skin changes on palpation to a firmer texture. As the peeling solution penetrates to the papillary dermis, the skin takes on an indurated, woody texture, and by mechanically moving the skin, the lines of facial expression become accentuated. As the peel penetrates into the reticular dermis, induration and hardness increase, and with further palpation and movement of the skin, the lines of facial expression are no longer discernible. *This obliteration of the lines of facial expression indicates the transition point between papillary and reticular dermal peeling and usually marks the end point of peeling.*

Return of Skin Color Following Resolution of Frosting

When TCA is applied to facial skin, the keratocoagulation of epidermal and dermal proteins causes the facial skin to appear white. As the TCA is neutralized by serum in the dermal vessels after application, the white appearance of the coagulated dermal protein resolves and the frosted appearance of facial skin changes to erythema. The length of time for the frosting to change to erythema is directly related to the depth of peel penetration. Peels that penetrate to the basement layer of the epidermis (pink/white frost) will assume an erythematous color approximately 10 to 15 minutes after application. Papillary dermal peels, which are associated with a uniform white frosting, will become erythematous in appearance 20 to 30 minutes following application. Reticular dermal peels associated with dense, opaque white frosting will assume an erythematous appearance between 40 to 60 minutes after application, whereas peels associated with deep dermal penetration and a grayish appearance are very slow to change color.

The return of color following peeling is a quantitative measurement of peel depth. As physicians gain experience with TCA peeling, they will learn to correlate clinical observations of frosting and turgor with color return to more accurately read the peel and be able to assess the degree of TCA penetration.

Methods to Increase TCA Penetration

TCA, unlike phenol, does not produce an all-or-none response. Low concentrations produce a light peel, whereas higher concentrations produce a deeper peel. Other methods of increasing TCA penetration include application of more coats of peeling solution, skin pretreatment with a keratolytic agent such as Jessner's solution (salicylic acid, lactic acid, and resorcinol), or mechanical abrasion with a gauze pad that is simultaneously used to apply the TCA solution. Obviously the degree of prepeel preparation with Retin-A will influence TCA penetration. In patients in whom peel preparation has been inadequate, peel penetration can be increased by chemical removal of the stratum corneum with Jessner's solution or mechanical removal of the stratum corneum by gauze abrasion.

DEEP PEELS

We prefer to perform reticular dermal TCA peels with the patient sedated to ensure greater comfort, allow adequate time to gauge the degree of frosting, and permit TCA application to the entire face rather than just regionally. We use a modified 40% to 45% TCA solution. Deep dermal peels require proper prepeel preparation to obtain consistent results. Peels at these depths are associated with longer recovery periods and more sustained postpeel erythema. Deep peels place the patient at greater risk of postpeel complications such as hyperpigmentation or hypertrophic scarring. When reticular dermal peels are performed, the margin between the desired depth of penetration and the potential for deep penetration must be understood. Accurately gauging the level of peel penetration is imperative to perform peels at this depth safely.

The quality of skin texture must be assessed carefully to ensure the success of reticular dermal peels. There is less margin of safety in patients with thin, dry skin, especially if their skin has been pretreated with Retin-A. Because the margin of safety in patients with thick, sebaceous skin is much greater, tyros would be well advised to choose patients with acne scarring for their initial experience with these deep dermal peels.

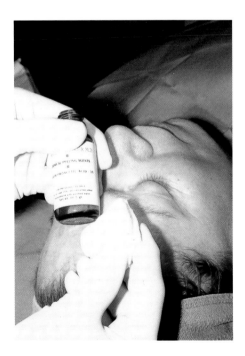

The technique of application for deep peels is similar to that described for medium-depth peels. We use 2 × 2 inch soaped sponges to mechanically apply the solution to the entire face in a single application. When peeling the lower lids, an assistant stabilizes the lid and applies the peeling solution with a semimoist Q-tip. Ophthalmic saline solution is always kept readily available should corneal lavage be necessary.

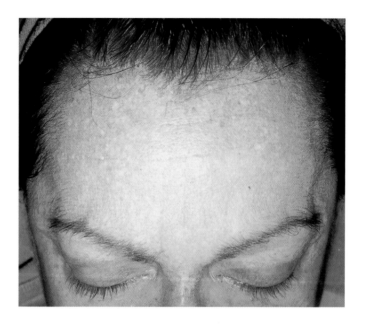

This patient had an upper reticular dermal chemical peel using a modified 40% TCA solution. The patient was sedated during peel application. The peeling solution has been applied uniformly to the forehead and the upper eyelids, although the pretarsal skin has not been treated to minimize postoperative eyelid edema.

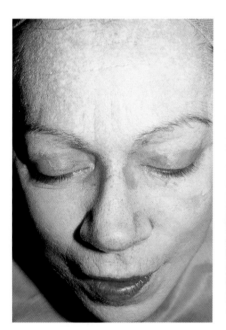 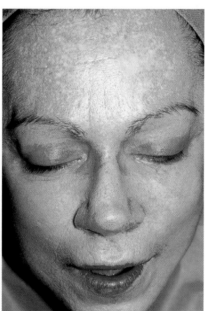 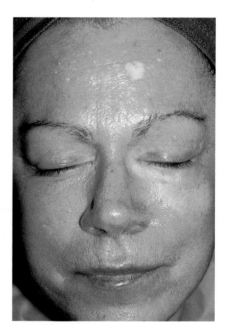

Note the uniform dense white frosting of facial skin immediately following TCA application. The patient is shown 20 minutes following the application of TCA to the forehead. At this time the forehead region, which was treated initially, is beginning to lose the dense frosting. One hour following peel application the frosting has resolved and the beginning of postpeel erythema is evident.

POSTPEEL CARE

Postpeel care will vary depending on the depth of peeling. Superficial peels involve a short recovery period, and moisturizers are all that is needed initially. After skin desquamation is completed, the patient may return to the prepeel skin routine consisting of Retin-A or glycolic acid and sunscreens.

Medium-depth peels require a more prolonged recovery and are associated with increased patient morbidity. Typically the normal daily routine of these patients is disrupted for approximately 5 to 7 days. During this period the skin appearance will change from erythematous to a profound brown, leathery appearance that correlates with desquamation of the epidermis and superficial dermis and reepithelialization.

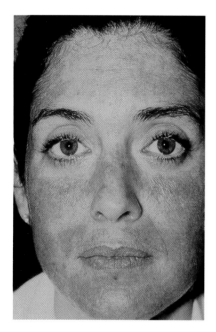 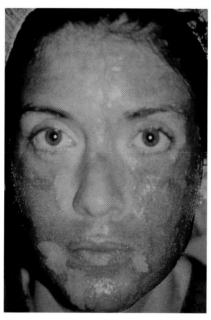 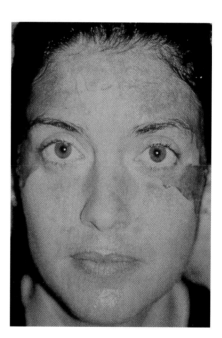

This patient had a 35% TCA peel. At 24 hours the initial postpeel erythema has changed to a mahogany color and the skin has a leathery texture. At 72 hours the desquamation appears more severe and the skin has a dense brown appearance. Four days after peeling much of the desquamated skin has exfoliated, revealing newly healed, fresh-appearing skin.

In the first week after a medium-depth peel patients are instructed to wash their faces four times a day with water and dilute hydrogen peroxide and then apply a petrolatum-based ointment (A & D ointment) or 1% hydrocortisone ointment. The skin commonly remains erythematous for a few days after reepithelialization, although patients can wear makeup once desquamation is complete. Seven to ten days following a medium-depth peel patients resume the application of Retin-A and hydroquinone, usually on alternating days. Once this regimen is tolerated they can resume daily applications for a few weeks to control postpeel hyperpigmentation. Sun avoidance and the use of sunscreens are important in the immediate postpeel period to prevent pigmentation.

Patient Instructions for TCA Peeling

TCA peeling is a procedure for rejuvenating facial skin. It restores a healthy, rosy glow to the skin, eliminates fine facial wrinkles, diminishes cross-hatching of the lower eyelids, and improves pigmented areas on the face and other regions of the body. TCA peeling is a multistage procedure. A second peel is typically performed 2 to 3 months after the first procedure to treat stubborn, coarse wrinkles such as those found on the forehead and upper lip. Complete removal of wrinkles and correction of facial pigmentation should not be anticipated. The degree of response to TCA peeling varies with each person.

Before Treatment

Preparation of the skin before peeling is critical to the success of the procedure. The skin is conditioned by applying Retin-A and hydroquinone for 4 to 6 weeks prior to peeling. You should apply these creams evenly over the entire area that is to be peeled. You will be given a prescription for these creams and instructions for its use. You must also use a sunscreen and moisturizer as part of the prepeel preparation.

Please wear no makeup whatsoever when you come to the office for the TCA peel. Wash your skin thoroughly with soap and water.

During Treatment

A degreasing agent will be applied by office personnel before the peeling process begins. When the TCA is applied, most individuals experience a flushing or reddening of the skin followed by a frosting of the skin that usually lasts for less than an hour. The slight stinging from the application lasts for 5 to 15 minutes. The staff will apply cool compresses and fan the area to help reduce the discomfort. Any minor discomfort will be over by the time you are discharged. Ointment will be applied following the procedure. Bandages are not necessary.

After Treatment

If you have been sedated, you will need to arrange for someone to drive you home from the office. There is usually very little discomfort associated with a TCA peel. Healing should be complete in 5 to 7 days, depending on the depth of the peel.

Initially the skin is slightly red. Eventually it becomes dry, often brown in pigmentation, and a crust will form. You usually will be instructed to apply a moisturizer such as A & D ointment or hydrocortisone ointment four times a day during the first 48 hours following the peel. After this, a standard facial moisturizer can be substituted for the greasier emulsions. You must use an ointment for 5 to 7 days until the crusting disappears. Twenty-four hours after treatment you may shower and gently wash the treated area with cool tap water. This daily routine is followed until the peeling is complete. Wash the face prior to each application of ointment. The redness of the skin may slightly intensify until the flaking is completed. The new skin should be evident within 5 to 7 days. By the end of 1 week the pink color should have faded to a light pink and have the appearance of a mild sunburn. The coloration usually fades completely within 2 to 3 weeks. You may use cosmetics as soon as the peeling process is finished.

A bleaching cream may be prescribed if you have pigmentation problems. The Retin-A routine may be resumed 10 days after treatment. Because the skin is sensitive after peeling, the Retin-A mixture should be lightly applied every other night until your skin is more tolerant of this regimen.

A sunscreen that has at least a 15 SPF (Shade-UVA) *must* be used for several weeks following the peel and at least until all the redness is gone. Establish the habit of applying the sunscreen in the morning before you leave your home.

Avoid intense facial expressions, bending, straining, or athletic activity until the areas are completely healed.

Irregular color changes, hyperpigmentation, and residual wrinkles after TCA peeling may sometimes occur. A second or third peel may be necessary to correct these problems. Scarring and numbness are rare possibilities but can occur. A bacterial or viral infection of the treated areas is rare but possible. If you have used Accutane in the past for the treatment of acne, please let us know.

Before your first peel, it is helpful to have the following items on hand:

- A & D ointment
- Hydrocortisone cream
- Moisturizer
- Sunscreen (Shade-UVA or any sunscreen with an SPF of at least 15)

All of these items may be purchased without a prescription.

Patient management following a deep peel is similar to that described for a medium-depth peel, although postpeel recovery is more prolonged. These patients commonly exhibit a greater degree of desquamation and postpeel erythema that can last for several weeks. Once reepithelialization has occurred, the Retin-A and hydroquinone skin treatment plan is resumed as noted above.

MULTIPLE PEELS

The long-term effect of TCA peeling varies from patient to patient; frequently it is necessary to repeat the peel. Superficial peels can be repeated at frequent intervals according to the needs and desires of the patient. Medium-depth and deep peels should be staged to allow adequate time for wound healing. We prefer to wait at least 2 to 3 months between medium-depth peels and usually longer than 3 months before repeating reticular dermal peels.

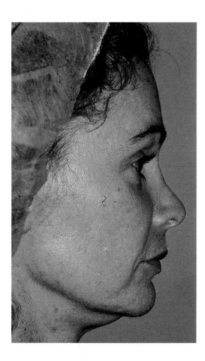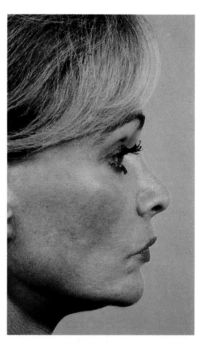

This patient had a face lift combined with a subsequent TCA peel. This case demonstrates how a medium-depth peel can enhance the overall results of surgical rejuvenation of the aging face.

RESULTS

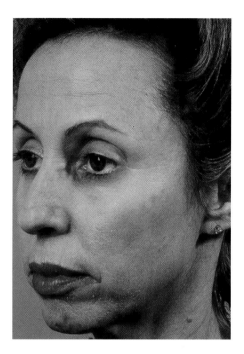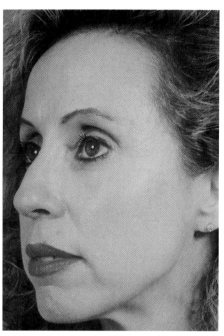

This patient has splotchy pigmentation secondary to actinic exposure and upper lip rhytides. Note the improvement following a 35% TCA peel and upper lip dermabrasion.

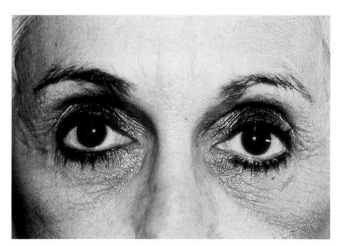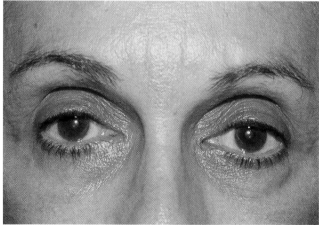

This patient was displeased with her periorbital rhytides and lower lid pigmentation. A 35% TCA peel was performed with good results.

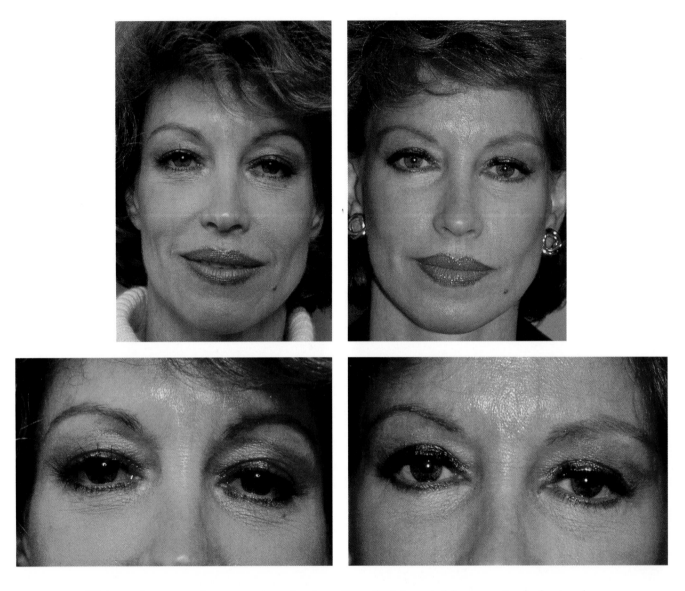

This patient sought treatment for her fine facial wrinkles, particularly in the periorbital region. She is shown 5 months after a 35% TCA peel.

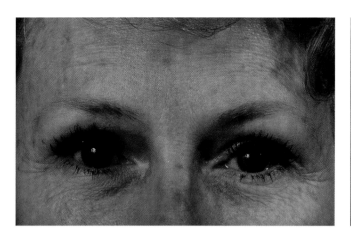
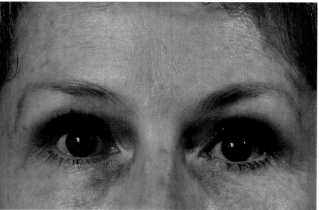

This patient clearly demonstrates the complementary effects of surgery and peeling. A blepharoplasty and TCA peel were performed.

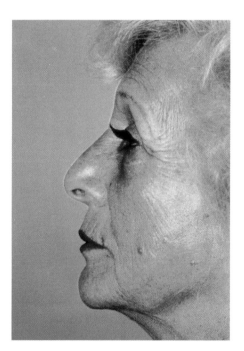
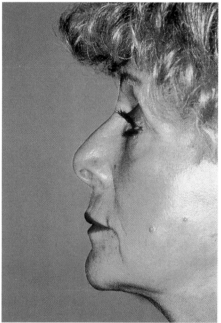

This patient shows evidence of both photoaging and intrinsic aging. The gravitational changes are manifest as nasolabial folds, jowling, and cervical obliquity. Actinic damage is exhibited by coarse and fine rhytides and splotchy facial hyperpigmentation. She is shown after a face lift followed by two medium-depth 35% TCA peels performed at 3-month intervals. Observe the improvement in the texture of her skin as well as a more uniform facial pigmentation and amelioration of facial wrinkling.

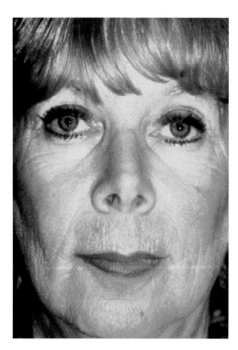 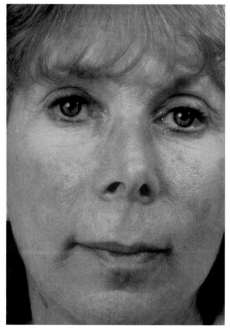

This patient reflects the gravitational changes of aging in association with coarse facial wrinkling. A face lift and upper lip dermabrasion were performed prior to a TCA peel. She is shown just before the second medium-depth peel was done to improve the remaining rhytides on her lower eyelid. This combination of treatment modalities adds precision to the ultimate postoperative result.

COMPLICATIONS
Postpeel Hyperpigmentation

The most common complication of TCA peeling we have seen in our practice is hyperpigmentation, which is usually caused by early sun exposure during the peripeel period when the skin is sensitive and reactive to UV light. The need for screens and avoidance of sun exposure until the skin is completely recovered from this chemical insult cannot be overstressed. Birth control pills and anticonvulsive medications have been associated with hyperpigmentation and should be discontinued should this troublesome complication develop.

Fortunately the pigment that forms is usually situated within the superficial epidermis and treatment is straightforward. Most patients with postpeel pigmentation will respond to nightly application of 0.1% Retin-A in combination with 4% hydroquinone applied twice daily. Alternatively, in patients who cannot tolerate Retin-A, twice-daily application of kojic acid and hydroquinone is useful for treating postinflammatory pigmentation. We recommend that our patients use these creams on a consistent basis over a 2- to 3-month period before any other treatment is considered. The majority of patients will respond to these creams as long as sun exposure is limited. If the pigmentation persists, a pretreatment skin regimen is begun in preparation for light to medium-depth peeling using a 25% to 35% TCA solution to the depth of the epidermal-dermal junction. This usually resolves the problem.

Scarring

Medium-depth and deep peels have been reported to cause hypertrophic scarring, but fortunately this has rarely occurred in our practice. As mentioned earlier, reticular dermal peels performed on well-retinized patients with thin, dry skin carry the greatest risk for deep dermal penetration of TCA. Scarring is most often seen in the perioral region and along the mandibular border. Peeling adjacent to surgically undermined skin and the previous use of isotretinoin (Accutane) may also lead to hypertrophic scarring. (Isotretinoin is an oral retinoid used in the treatment of acne that suppresses adnexal structures.) Postpeel scarring has been noted in patients who have discontinued isotretinoin for as long as 24 months before the peel. As a general policy, we avoid deep peeling in patients who have been using isotretinoin until they have discontinued its use for at least 1 year. Once these patients develop normal oil secretion, it is usually safe to consider peeling.

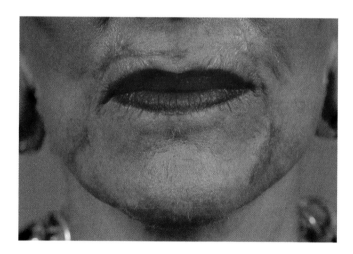

Depth of penetration does not always correlate with neocollagen formation and the improvement of facial rhytides. We have been consistently disappointed with the failure of TCA peeling to improve perioral rhytides even when carried to the level of the deep reticular dermis. This patient is seen following a 50% TCA peel performed in another office. Note the hypertrophic scarring in the perioral region in conjunction with the persistence of perioral rhytides despite the obvious deep penetration of the TCA.

Injectable corticosteroids and silicone pressure taping are used to treat hypertrophic scarring. Surgical revision or dermabrasion can be done following scar maturation to improve the cosmetic appearance of these scars.

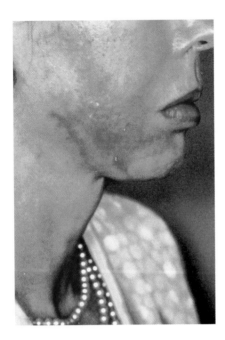

This patient developed hypertrophic scarring of the cheek and perioral region following a reticular dermal TCA peel at an outlying clinic. Controlling the depth of the TCA peeling agent is the key to safe, consistent results and avoidance of scarring.

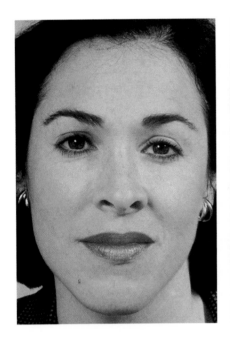
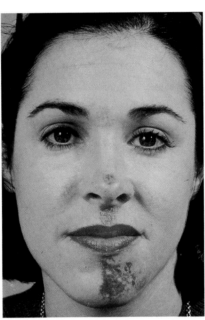
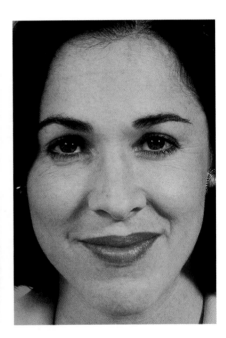

This patient exhibits delayed healing following 35% TCA peeling taken to the level of the reticular dermis. Two weeks after peeling persistent eschar signified delayed healing in the perioral region. Six weeks after peeling reepithelialization has occurred without hypertrophic scarring. Patients who exhibit late reepithelialization following any form of resurfacing should be managed conservatively with topical ointments and frequent observation. If hypertrophic scarring develops, it should be dealt with aggressively in the early stages with low-dose intralesional steroid injections.

Herpes Simplex Infection

Herpes simplex infection may be aggravated by peeling to any depth. We ask all patients if they have a history of herpes infection. Those patients with a positive history can be treated prophylactically with 400 mg of acyclovir (Zovirax) three times daily beginning the day before the peel and continuing for 4 days after peeling. Valacyclovir (Valtrex), 500 mg twice a day, is another useful agent for preventing postpeel herpes infection. If a patient who has not been treated prophylactically develops a postpeel herpes infection, acyclovir or valacyclovir is started immediately. For severe infections, this regimen can be increased to 800 mg three times a day as clinically required. Although herpes infections are common following peeling, residual scarring is rare if promptly treated.

CONCLUDING THOUGHTS

TCA peels perhaps have the broadest indications for treating a wide range of dermatologic conditions and are applicable to a diverse patient population. No other treatment modality has such variability in application, ranging from superficial refresher peels to deep reticular dermal penetration. The learning curve in performing TCA peels is prolonged because of the numerous factors that affect peel penetration and posttreatment results.

The key to successful TCA peeling is perfecting a pretreatment regimen that can be consistently applied as well as proper patient evaluation. The ability to control peel depth is essential to consistent results and minimal postpeel sequelae.

REFERENCES

Ayres S. Dermal changes following application of chemical cauterants to aging skin (superficial chemosurgery). Arch Dermatol 82:578, 1960.

Ayres S. Superficial chemosurgery in treating aging skin. Arch Dermatol 85:125, 1962.

Baker TJ, Stuzin JM. Chemical peeling and dermabrasion. In McCarthy JG, ed. Plastic Surgery. Philadelphia: WB Saunders, 1990, p 748.

Baker TJ, Gordon HL, Stuzin JM. Chemical peeling (phenol and trichloroacetic acid) and dermabrasion. In Surgical Rejuvenation of the Face, 2nd ed. St. Louis: Mosby, 1996, p 45.

Brody HJ. Medium-depth chemical peeling of the skin: A variation of superficial chemosurgery. Adv Dermatol 3:205, 1988.

Brody HJ. Variations and comparisons in medium-depth chemical peeling. J Dermatol Surg Oncol 15:953, 1989.

Brody HJ. Chemical Peeling. St. Louis: Mosby–Year Book, 1992.

Brody HJ, Hailey CW. Medium-depth chemical peeling of the skin: A variation of superficial chemosurgery. J Dermatol Surg Oncol 12:1268, 1986.

Collins PS. The chemical peel. Clin Dermatol 5:57, 1987.

Collins PS. Trichloroacetic acid peels revisited. J Dermatol Surg Oncol 15:933, 1989.

Monheit GD. The Jessner's + TCA peel: A medium-depth chemical peel. J Dermatol Surg Oncol 15:945, 1989.

Resnik SS. Chemical peeling with trichloroacetic acid. J Dermatol Surg Oncol 10:549, 1984.

Resnik SS. Chemical peeling with trichloroacetic acid. In Roenigk H, Roenigk R, eds. Dermatologic Surgery: Principles and Practice. New York: Marcel Dekker, 1989, pp 979-995.

Resnik SS, Lewis LA, Cohen BH. Trichloroacetic acid peeling. Cutis 17:127, 1976.

Rubin MG. Manual of Chemical Peels: Superficial and Medium Depth. Philadelphia: JB Lippincott,
1995.

Stagnone JJ. Chemical peeling and chemabrasion. In Epstein E, ed. Skin Surgery, 6th ed. Philadelphia: WB Saunders, 1987, p 412.

Steman SJ, Tromovitch TA, Glogau RG. Cosmetic Dermatologic Surgery, 2nd ed. St. Louis:
Mosby–Year Book, 1990, pp 35-58.

Stuzin JM, Baker TJ, Gordon HL. Treatment of photoaging: Facial chemical peeling (phenol and trichloroacetic acid) and dermabrasion. Clin Plast Surg 20:9, 1993.

Wolfort FG, Dalton WE, Hoopes JE. Chemical peel with trichloroacetic acid. Br J Plast Surg 25:333,
1972.

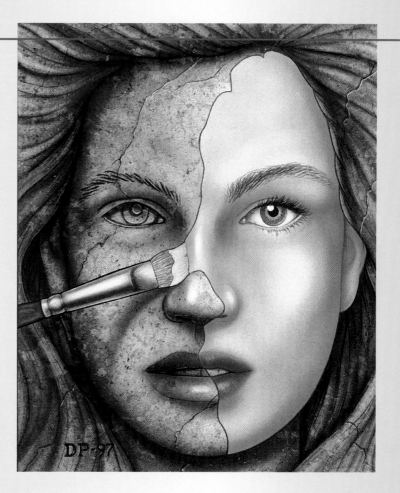

Phenol Peels

Phenol, the prototypical deep chemical peeling agent, produces profound results. The dramatic clinical and histologic effects are exceptionally durable. The contrast with unpeeled skin is remarkable even after 20 years. When applied to the skin, phenol induces a controlled, predictable chemical injury—a partial-thickness chemical burn—that on healing results in smoother, more youthful-appearing skin. The long-term effect is most likely attributable to the consistent depth of penetration into the upper reticular dermis resulting in the consistent formation of a new stratified collagen layer. Phenol is the standard against which other treatment modalities for aged and actinically damaged skin are measured. It is a safe, effective treatment for removing fine and coarse facial wrinkling and irregular facial pigmentation localized to the dermis and for ablating actinic keratoses.

This deep peeling agent, however, is not without its drawbacks. Unlike TCA peels that cause more limited morbidity and can be used to treat a broad range of individuals, phenol peels are associated with a more prolonged recovery and a significant bleaching action, thereby limiting their application and appeal. Phenol peels are indicated for a limited group of patients, especially in the treatment of regional problems, largely because its bleaching effect can produce an obvious line of demarcation between treated and untreated skin. These peels are ideal for treating patients with coarse facial wrinkling and significant perioral rhytides. Similarly, in patients with facial hyperpigmentation localized to the dermis, the uniform lightening obtained with phenol peeling produces consistent results.

Other deep resurfacing agents such as dermabrasion and the UltraPulse CO_2 laser offer alternative methods for treatment of coarse facial rhytides. Dermabrasion is highly effective in the perioral region and has less of a bleaching effect than phenol. It has more limited applicability in the treatment of facial rhytides and cannot be used in the treatment periorbital rhytides. Laser resurfacing is replacing phenol because it produces fewer changes in facial pigmentation, making it applicable to a broad spectrum of patients and an ideal agent for regional resurfacing. However, even with multiple passes of the laser at high energy levels, laser resurfacing is often not as effective in the treatment of coarse rhytides as phenol. Posttreatment recovery for laser patients is similar to that following a phenol peel.

HISTOLOGIC CHANGES

Phenol produces a controlled chemical injury that extends through the epidermis into the superficial dermis. Epithelial appendages are the sites of healing and regeneration after chemical peeling. Epidermal regeneration begins 48 hours after the peel and is usually complete by 7 to 10 days. The cells of the epidermis show a return of vertical polarity, stain more evenly, and are more uniform in size and shape. Melanocytes remain within the basement membrane and contain evenly dispersed, fine pigment granules. This reorganization eliminates the tendency to form irregular local pigmentations and lentigines.

Dermal regeneration begins 1 to 2 weeks after peeling and is nearly complete by 3 months. The postpeel dermis exhibits a profound reorganization consisting of horizontally arranged, compact, parallel bundles of collagen. A network of fine elastic fibers courses through this zone, often conforming to the collagen configuration. This newly formed collagen-elastic network within the papillary dermis is responsible for the smoother, fuller, and more turgid appearance of postpeel skin. Although the process of aging continues, the histologic changes and the clinical improvements produced by phenol peeling are long lasting. Indeed, biopsies performed on peeled and adjacent unpeeled skin 20 years after treatment confirm the longevity of the results.

Phenol is a keratocoagulant that originally was used in carbolic acid as a disinfectant. Because of the extreme keratocoagulation phenol produces, its use and depth of penetration differ from that of TCA. Since it evokes an all-or-none response, a low concentration of phenol does not necessarily produce a light peel. Conversely, a high concentration cannot be expected to produce a deeper peel. Actually, the opposite appears to be true. High concentrations of phenol are associated with more rapid and complete keratin coagulation in the epidermis. The resulting coagulant layer acts as a barrier to further penetration of the acid and lessens its effect on the dermis. Histologic studies have demonstrated that 100% concentrations of phenol produce 35% to 50% less penetration than a 50% phenol solution. Therefore increasing the phenol concentration may increase the risk of systemic toxicity but will not improve the clinical result.

TOXICOLOGY

Phenol is absorbed through the skin, detoxified in the liver, and excreted by the kidneys. A toxic dose of phenol absorbed systemically injures both the liver and kidneys and can depress the respiratory centers and myocardium. Studies have shown that only small blood levels of phenol are absorbed systemically following topical full-face peeling, indicating that the small volume of phenol used during facial peeling poses little risk of causing a systemic toxic reaction.

Of more concern to a physician performing phenol chemical peels is the possibility of rapid phenol absorption. Truppman and Ellenby noted a high incidence of cardiac arrhythmias when phenol was applied to over 50% of the facial surface in less than 30 minutes. When application over the same area was increased to 60 minutes, arrhythmias were avoided. Presumably, higher levels of phenol absorption can produce myocardial irritability. The arrhythmias observed range from atrial tachycardia to premature ventricular contractions. We have found in our large series of patients that electrocardiographic changes following phenol application are rare, especially if the phenol is applied regionally over a period of 1 or 2 hours. As a result, all patients undergoing phenol peeling should be monitored electrocardiographically and have an intravenous line in place. Medication and personnel to treat cardiac arrhythmias should be readily available.

INDICATIONS

The strong bleaching action associated with phenol chemical peel makes proper patient selection crucial for achieving satisfactory results. Patients with fair complexions and little sun exposure are better candidates than those with darker complexions. In general regional peeling can be performed in fair-complexioned patients, whereas patients with olive complexions usually require a full-face peel to minimize the contrast between peeled and unpeeled skin. In a dark-skinned individual a phenol peel may result in a distinct line of demarcation between treated and untreated skin. Red-haired, freckled patients with fine wrinkles around the eyes and mouth are also poor candidates for regional phenol peeling because an obvious line of demarcation will result after peeling. Although the peeling removes the wrinkles, it also bleaches the pale freckles. Even if the peeling is restricted to a small area of the face such as the upper lip, it will create a disturbing color disparity between the new freckle-free white lip and the rest of the face. There is no satisfactory method to "feather" the line of demarcation in these types of patients, and the only solution is to perform a full-face peel so that the line of demarcation between the face and neck is less obvious. Proper patient selection for phenol peeling will ensure that one problem is not solved at the risk of creating another one. If the line of demarcation at the junction between treated and untreated skin is obvious, the patient will have to wear makeup to camouflage it.

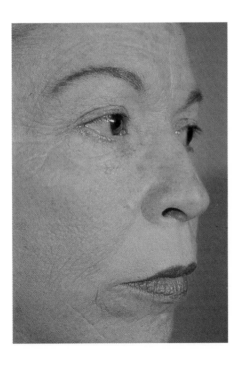

Patients with Fitzpatrick type I skin commonly have red hair, are freckled, and have visible coarse and fine rhytides from actinic exposure. Because of the effects of photoaging, the skin of these individuals will commonly have a brownish hue even though they are actually extremely fair. These types of individuals are poor candidates for regional phenol peeling since they will usually develop severe hypopigmentation. In this patient the line of demarcation between treated and untreated skin is extreme. This patient has the alternative of having a full-face phenol peel (which will make her extremely white) or using camouflaging makeup.

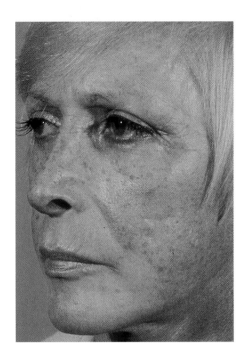

Patients with Fitzpatrick type II skin are quite fair but will usually develop a mottled complexion in response to significant actinic exposure. When considering regional phenol peeling, it is important to visualize how the bleaching effect of phenol will contrast with adjacent, untreated photodamaged skin. A perioral phenol peel that extended into this patient's lower cheek produced an obvious line of demarcation that is difficult to conceal with makeup. The only solution to this difficult problem is to peel the rest of her face, although a visible line of demarcation between treated facial skin and untreated cervical skin will remain.

Thick, oily skin may respond less favorably to a phenol peel. Natural skin oils seem to reduce the permeability and effectiveness of the peeling solution, and the skin will have a greater tendency to develop areas of spotty hypopigmentation.

Men, with few exceptions, are poor candidates because they shun the use of cosmetics. In addition, the thick skin of males usually does not respond as well as the thinner skin of women.

Phenol peels are probably not the best option for black and Oriental patients since many of these patients will exhibit blotchy hyperpigmentation with areas of hypopigmentation. For these patients, a TCA peel may be a better solution, especially in conjunction with a consistent prepeel regimen. When a patient with a darker complexion continues to insist on a phenol peel despite the obvious line of demarcation that is most certain to occur, we show her a photograph of a patient with similar skin who has had a phenol peel so that she can more realistically assess whether she will be satisfied with the results. Some women with numerous fine wrinkles or disorders of facial pigmentation are willing to accept the line of demarcation, especially if this line can be hidden just caudal to the mandibular border.

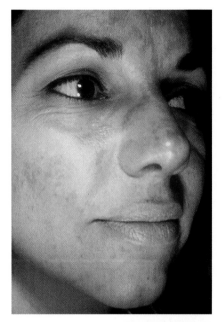 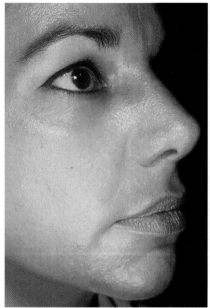

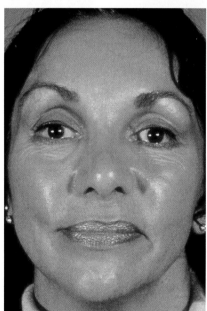

Patients with Fitzpatrick types III and IV skin are usually not ideal candidates for phenol peeling. Nonetheless, we have successfully performed full-face peels in these individuals with good results even though we believe they are not ideal candidates for regional peeling. This patient has an olive, Mediterranean complexion. Her deep dermal blotchy pigmentation is secondary to birth control pill use and actinic exposure. She is shown 1 year after a full-face peel to eliminate the hyperpigmentation. The line of demarcation is hidden just inferior to the mandibular border. Sixteen years after the phenol peel the facial pigmentation has not recurred and she exhibits minimal facial wrinkling despite continued sun exposure.

Phenol is effective for treating fine and coarse facial wrinkling and blotchy skin pigmentation caused by pregnancy, birth control pills, chronic solar exposure, and various dermatitides. The most common regional application is the treatment of perioral wrinkling. Spot applications of pure phenol can also be used to treat individual lentigines on the dorsum of the hands and fingers to predictably eradicate these signs of aging. Light and medium-depth TCA peels may be more effective for treating more generalized "age spots" of the forearm and hands so common in elderly patients.

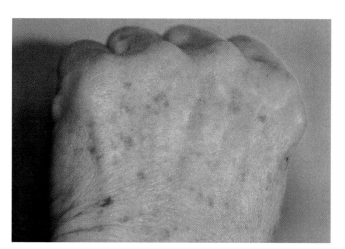 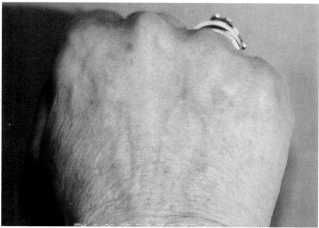

Spot peeling of lentigines of the hand with phenol is quite effective. In this patient spot peeling was performed on the right hand while the left hand was untreated. It is well accepted that TCA peeling can remove the superficial pigmentation of aged hands and forearms; however, we have also had success in using phenol for even deeper pigmentation spots. Phenol application to the entire dorsum of the hand is obviously contraindicated since it could result in catastrophic hypertrophic scarring.

Precancerous lesions as a consequence of radiation (solar) exposure are amenable to treatment with phenol peeling. The regeneration of dysplastic epithelium following chemical peeling is an added benefit in patients who present with sun damage and actinic keratoses and who undergo peeling for facial wrinkling.

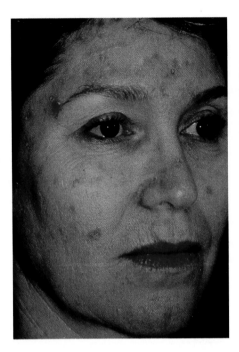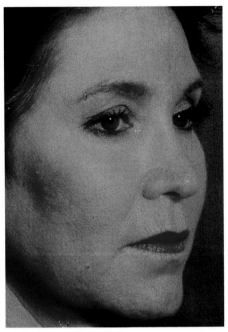

Patients with Fitzpatrick type II skin and significant actinic damage commonly develop epithelial dysplasia, multiple actinic keratoses, and incipient basal cell carcinomas. The regeneration of a normal epithelium following phenol peeling also produces desirable results. In this patient a phenol peel eliminated multiple actinic keratoses and improved facial wrinkling.

Phenol peels are effective in patients with superficial acne scarring, but patients with deep acne scarring with associated facial pitting and cysts will likely be poor candidates. Capillary hemangiomas, facial telangiectasias, port-wine stains, changes in pigmentation resulting from thermal burns, and hypertrophied scars also will not respond to this treatment.

Phenol peeling should not be used to treat rhytides or pigmentation of the neck, thorax, or extremities. Attempts at peeling these areas with phenol have resulted in hypertrophic scarring, and phenol toxicity may occur because of the large area to be treated.

TECHNIQUE

Phenol peeling should be performed in a hospital or ambulatory surgery facility. Sedation is required before and after full-face peeling, but the need for sedation and monitoring is not as pressing in cases of regional or spot facial peeling. Our patients scheduled for full-face phenol peels are given 5 to 10 mg oral diazepam on arrival. This is supplemented with intravenous meperidine prior to phenol application and as needed in the postpeel period. Midazolam also can be administered in incremental doses to enhance sedation and for its overall amnestic effects.

Experienced personnel must be available to monitor the patient for 1 to 2 days after peeling because of the anticipated eyelid edema. An intravenous catheter is placed, and the patient is monitored with electrocardiographic and pulse oximetry equipment.

Skin Preparation and Degreasing

In contrast to other deep resurfacing procedures such as TCA and laser resurfacing and dermabrasion, we do not pretreat patients who are to have a phenol peel with Retin-A. We do not know if Retin-A would increase phenol penetration as it does with TCA and are concerned about the depth of penetration with pretreatment. Historically, the consistent results obtained with phenol have made a preoperative skin care regimen unnecessary.

The night before the procedure the patient is instructed to thoroughly cleanse her face to remove all traces of makeup. Prior to peeling the patient's skin is cleansed with liquid soap and water and completely dried. All traces of makeup and surface oils must be removed from the skin to enhance the peeling process; diethyl ether or any other organic solvent such as acetone can be used for this purpose. If neither of these is available, isopropyl alcohol can be used. The removal of surface oils prior to phenol application is extremely important because inadequately degreased skin can lead to uneven peel penetration.

Formula Preparation

We have used the following formula for many years with safe and reliable results.

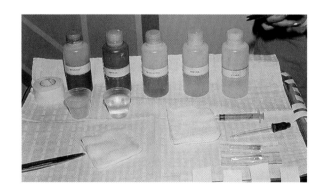

Baker-Gordon Formula
3 ml USP liquid phenol
2 ml tap water
8 drops liquid soap
3 drops croton oil

The phenol comes as a liquid solution in a concentration of approximately 88% phenol. Initially we recommended that distilled water be used as a diluent, but we now believe that tap water works as well. Liquid soap is used to saponify the mixture. We use Septicol for this purpose, but any liquid soap will do. Croton oil, extracted from the seeds of *Croton tiglium*, serves as a vesicant. Although this ingredient may be difficult to find, some pharmaceutical houses in larger cities continue to stock this ancient medication. If croton oil is unavailable, it can be eliminated, although we believe croton oil enhances the mixture's keratolytic and penetrating action and produces a more profound result.

Rather than entrusting a pharmacist, we prepare a fresh batch of the chemical mixture prior to each use. The ingredients do not readily combine and must be stirred vigorously before each application.

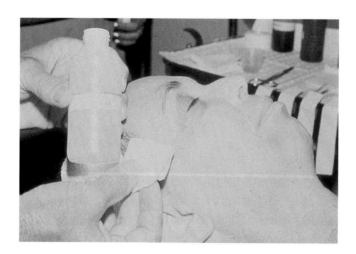

Prior to phenol application the face is thoroughly washed with soap and water and then all surface oils removed with ether or acetone.

Application

The peeling mixture is applied to the skin with a cotton-tipped applicator that is damp but not overly moist to eliminate dripping and streaking of areas such as the neck that are not to be peeled. Lightly rolling the applicator onto a piece of gauze absorbs the excess liquid and helps avoid this problem. When the eyelids are to be treated, the applicator must be nearly dry to prevent the phenol from contacting the cornea and conjunctiva. We keep a supply of sterile water available for irrigation in case of accidental eye contact.

The formula is painted on evenly to ensure complete coverage of the face and penetration into each wrinkle. Areas missed during the initial application will be glaringly evident later on. When the formula is applied to the skin, it immediately turns a frosty grayish white. The patient experiences a burning sensation that usually lasts a few minutes and then subsides because of the local anesthetic property of phenol. The solution should be applied slowly to minimize the burning sensation accompanying the peeling process and to avoid rapid phenol absorption. The application is completed over the course of 1 to 2 hours. The solution is applied regionally to the face. Applicators are changed frequently so that the formula on the applicator mixes with as little of the skin oil as possible; an average of 8 to 10 applicators will be used for a full-face peel.

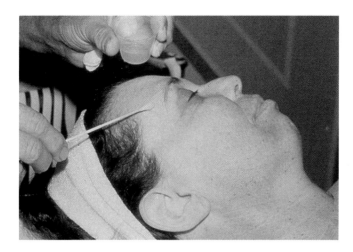

We prefer to apply the phenol mixture as a regional application and usually apply the peeling agent to the forehead first. The phenol is applied into the hairline close to and even into the eyebrows to minimize the line of demarcation where the peeling stops. The peeling agent will not affect hair growth in these areas and will not cause alopecia.

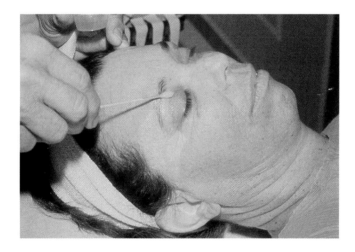

When treating the upper eyelid, phenol is also applied to the eyebrow and preseptal upper lid skin. The peel usually stops at the upper border of the tarsus to minimize postpeel eyelid edema. The upper eyelid is treated down to the tarsal plate, but generally the ciliary margin is avoided to help reduce the immediate postpeel edema. The pretarsal skin usually does not require peeling. The upper eyelid skin can be taped, but no tape is applied directly over the eyebrows.

Within 20 to 30 minutes the malar region and cheeks, including the lower eyelids, are treated. When the lower lids are peeled, the skin is moistened to within 3 mm of the lid margins. An assistant holds the upper eyelids open to prevent blinking until each of the lower lids has been treated, blotted, and allowed to air dry.

The solution is painted on the lower third of the face to just below the mandibular border since it is the least conspicuous place for the inevitable line of demarcation between treated and untreated skin. Prior to beginning the peel it is helpful to mark the area caudal to the mandibular border with the patient in an upright position to ensure that this peel line is accurately positioned. In the perioral area care is taken to paint the formula to the vermilion border and preferably slightly onto it so that there is not even the slightest rim of untreated skin around the lips. One of the most common prepeel complaints of women is that lipstick bleeds into the lip lines. Application along the vermilion removes these troublesome vertical wrinkles of the upper lip, especially the small ones radiating from the vermilion border. Small wrinkles of the earlobes can also be eradicated.

Occlusive Dressings

After each region of the face has been completely covered with the peeling solution, an occlusive dressing is applied. Numerous studies have demonstrated that use of an occlusive dressing increases the depth of phenol penetration. The dressing probably prevents evaporation of the phenol solution and promotes tissue maceration, thereby inducing greater penetration. Two types of dressing can be used: a waterproof mask of adhesive tape or a Vaseline occlusive dressing.

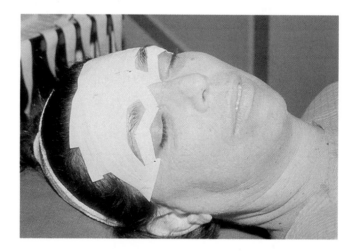

When a waterproof tape mask is used as an occlusive dressing, it is immediately applied after each region of the face has been covered with the peeling solution. Although the tape is applied to the preseptal skin of the upper eyelid, note that it is not applied directly over the eyebrow.

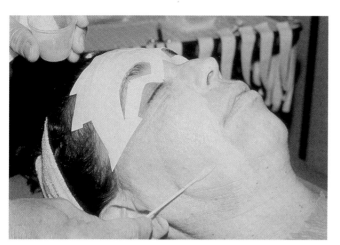
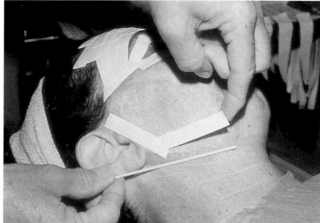

After the forehead is treated, phenol is applied regionally to the adjacent cheek. Once the peel is completed, waterproof tape is applied to the treated region.

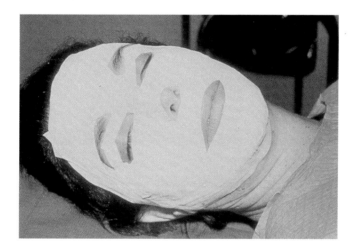

The only areas of the face left uncovered after treatment and taping are the eyebrows, pretarsal skin of the upper lid, nasal tip, and upper and lower vermilion.

When a waterproof mask of adhesive tape is used, it is applied directly to the skin. Only the eyes, eyebrows, nostrils, and mouth remain exposed. Short pieces of tape are used because they more easily conform to the facial curves. When first applied, the tape may not adhere well. As the natural body heat warms the adhesive and early edema occurs, the tape will become more adherent. The tape should not be applied tightly. Improper tape application can result in folded or pleated skin that is not in contact with the tape and will result in skin that is streaked and uneven in texture and color. After the treated area is covered with strips of ½-inch tape, a second layer of 1-inch strips is placed over the first to reinforce the mask and ensure total coverage. Approximately 20 to 30 minutes after the tape mask is applied, the burning sensation returns, this time with greater intensity and for a longer period. Analgesics help reduce patient discomfort and narcotics are usually necessary.

In our experience occlusive taping maintains the greatest concentration of phenol at the skin surface and produces a more profound, long-lasting peel. However, taping has several disadvantages, including increased patient discomfort, particularly during tape removal, and preventing the physician from evaluating the wound. After the tape mask is removed, the skin is generally treated with an application of thymol iodide, which dries the wounds and forms a superficial eschar. Although wound healing following thymol iodide application is predictable, drying of the skin followed by separation of the crusts from the face after desquamation and healing may be painful for the patient. The advantages of enhancing the depth of penetration of the phenol mixture must be weighed against the increased morbidity associated with tape mask occlusion.

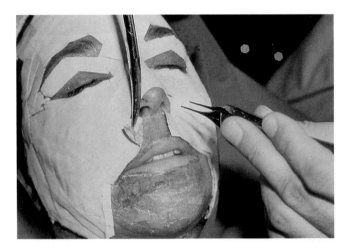

We typically remove the tape mask 48 hours following phenol application. The patient has been medicated with an oral analgesic agent. The tape is removed in sections, revealing the underlying desquamated wound.

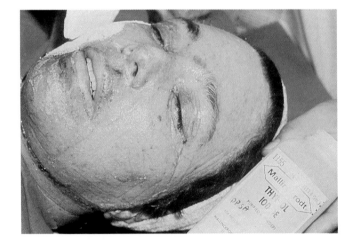

The open wounds are then dusted with thymol iodide.

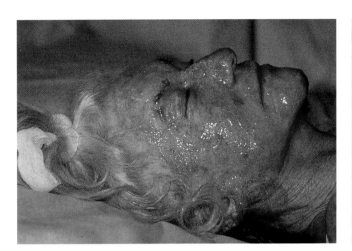
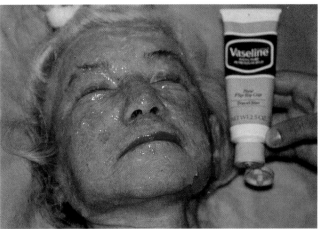

An alternative to occlusive taping is use of a Vaseline occlusive dressing. In patients with moderate actinic damage we favor the use of a Vaseline occlusive dressing as opposed to a tape mask. Similar to tape application, the Vaseline is applied to each region after regional phenol application. The Vaseline must not be applied to adjacent untreated skin since this will interfere with the phenol application in this area. At the end of the procedure a final layer of Vaseline is applied evenly to the entire face. The Vaseline dressing lubricates the wound, tends to prevent phenol evaporation, and thereby increases phenol penetration. Wound lubrication is continued throughout the early postpeel period with an oily, petrolatum-based ointment such as A & D ointment. Gentle washing of the peeled area with cool tap water is initiated on the first day after the peel, and this routine of lavage followed by application of an ointment continues until wound healing is completed 5 to 7 days later. At no time is the wound allowed to desiccate.

Although the Vaseline occlusive dressing produces a less dramatic result than tape occlusion, it also avoids the disadvantages associated with taping. For this reason, we have used tape dressings less frequently in the past several years and now tend to favor the Vaseline occlusive mask. The occlusion provided by the thick layer of jelly has proved to be almost as effective as the tape mask and the results parallel those achieved with tape. The occlusive dressing is of the greatest benefit in the hours immediately following phenol application. It acts as a mechanical barrier to enhance the results of the chemical peel.

This method has several advantages. The patient experiences less discomfort, the wound beneath the mask can be evaluated more easily, and the streaking that can result from uneven tape application is eliminated. Eschar formation and crust separation are avoided by the liberal use of lubricants such as A & D ointment.

We currently use Vaseline occlusive dressings for all peels to treat facial pigmentation problems and fine facial wrinkling. We reserve tape occlusion for difficult clinical problems that require a greater degree of penetration. Tape occlusion is therefore used to treat patients with coarse wrinkling and a "weather-beaten" appearance to obtain a more profound result.

In summary, phenol application produces an all-or-none response, and unlike TCA peeling, varying the concentration of phenol will not necessarily produce a lighter or more profound result. The method we have found most useful in controlling phenol penetration is the use of an occlusive dressing. An adhesive tape mask produces the deepest phenol penetration and provides the most consistent results for coarse rhytides. This must be counterbalanced by increased patient morbidity. If no dressing is used, phenol penetration will be significantly decreased. This may be acceptable for fine rhytides but is less predictable when coarse rhytides are present. Use of a Vaseline occlusive dressing is an acceptable compromise and allows the physician to predictably improve coarse rhytides while also decreasing the morbidity in the immediate postpeel period.

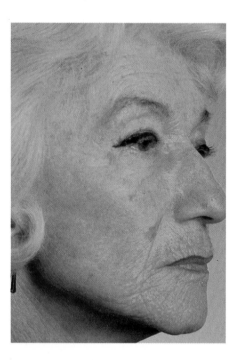 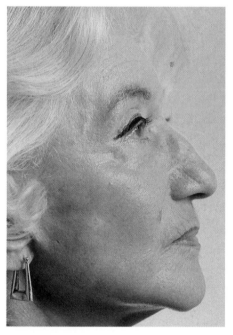

This patient has significant actinic damage with coarse and fine facial rhytides. Observe the improved appearance following a full-face phenol peel and use of a Vaseline occlusive dressing.

BUFFERED PHENOL SOLUTIONS

Many phenol solutions are now formulated in various concentrations to enhance or limit penetration. These different formulas, the so-called buffered phenol solutions, are reported to cause less hypopigmentation than the Baker-Gordon formula. The use of croton oil appears to be particularly important in enhancing or limiting phenol penetration. Formulas that use lower concentrations of croton oil produce less phenol penetration, thereby limiting postpeel hypopigmentation.

We have limited experience using buffered phenol formulas but have examined patients who have had buffered phenol peels. It is our impression that while the bleaching effect produced by these solutions is less than traditional formulas, the improvement of coarse facial rhytides is inconsistent. Obviously limiting phenol penetration will decrease postpeel hypopigmentation, but it will also reduce neocollagen formation. In our opinion alternative options such as laser resurfacing or dermabrasion are perhaps better suited for patients likely to develop unacceptable postpeel hypopigmentation.

POSTPEEL CARE

The intravenous line is left in place for the first 5 or 6 hours after the phenol peel to administer sedatives to blunt the burning sensation. The intensity of the burning varies from patient to patient. Some will complain bitterly, whereas others require little or no medication. After 6 or 8 hours this burning sensation subsides and discomfort can be managed with oral medications.

Theoretically, patients can ambulate in the immediate postpeel period; however, their mobility is often limited by eyelid edema. Edema is greatest during the first 6 to 12 hours after treatment. For some, eyelid edema is severe enough to blur vision. Elevation of the head of the bed helps minimize edema. Experienced personnel should be in attendance to reassure the patient.

When an adhesive mask is applied, the patient is instructed to talk as little as possible so that the tape remains adherent around the lips. Patients take liquids through a straw and are encouraged to drink large quantities of fluid.

The mask is removed in 24 to 48 hours, depending on the amount of edema. Medication can be given when the adhesive tape mask is removed. Some epithelium will adhere to the undersurface of the waterproof adhesive tape as the mask is removed. Patches of loose epithelium will also remain over the face; no attempt should be made to remove them.

The newly uncovered skin has the appearance of a uniform superficial second-degree chemical burn. The unprepared patient may be alarmed by this appearance. The skin surface is edematous and moist and may have punctate hemorrhages and scattered islands of epithelium. It may be covered with a thin layer of loose detritus consisting of necrotic epithelium and coagulated exudate. Cleansing the eyelashes and corners of the eyes with a cotton applicator and, if necessary, hydrogen peroxide makes the patient more comfortable. If no mask is applied, there is less edema, which simplifies management of the peeled areas. When a tape mask is not used, the wounds are simply washed thoroughly with tap water or a dilute solution of tap water and peroxide four times a day and then covered with a thin layer of A & D ointment. This routine of wound cleansing and ointment application is continued until reepithelialization is complete. The physician should check patients frequently during the immediate peripeel period until they can adequately care for their wounds.

Reepithelialization is the hallmark of wound healing and usually occurs 7 to 10 days following phenol application. After this time the skin will appear erythematous, but the edema should have subsided almost completely. The patient is instructed to continue washing her face gently and lubricate the skin with greasy moisturizers, Crisco, cocoa butter, or hydrocortisone creams. Petrolatum-based ointments such as A & D ointment are discontinued after reepithelialization is completed. Pain is unusual after this period of time, but some patients may experience discomfort, especially at night. Itching commonly occurs following reepithelialization and often will persist until the postpeel erythema has faded. If itching is symptomatic, patients are advised to apply ice-water compresses frequently. Antihistamines are often useful in this period of healing.

Depending on the rate of healing, at the end of 10 to 15 days the patient is allowed to use cosmetics. Specific instructions are given regarding exposure of the newly peeled areas to sunlight. Sunscreens must be used as soon as the skin is able to tolerate these protective agents, generally in 12 to 14 days. The erythematous color persists for as long as 10 to 12 weeks, but in rare cases it may take as long as 6 months. In patients with persistent erythema we have found that topically applied mild cortisone creams may hasten resolution of the redness. The patient is instructed to continue daily application of sunscreens even after healing is complete. She is also advised that her skin will never tan normally again and sun exposure should be avoided. Excessive unprotected exposure to the sun may cause blotchy skin, necessitating treatment for postpeel hyperpigmentation. If this troublesome problem develops, the patient should be immediately started on a program of Retin-A and hydroquinone skin care. Usually postpeel hyperpigmentation is limited to the superficial epidermis and dermis and will respond to skin care alone, although occasionally medium-depth TCA peeling will be required to alleviate this problem.

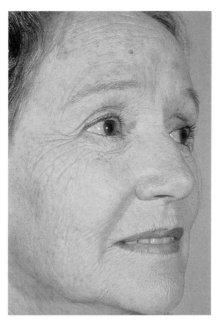

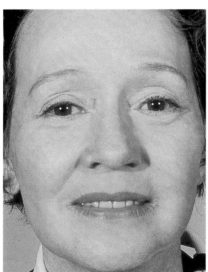
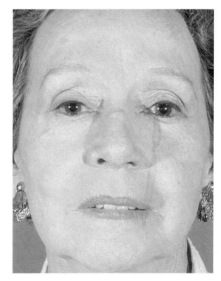

This patient exhibits coarse and fine rhytides secondary to chronic sun exposure. Note the elimination of facial wrinkling 6 months following a phenol peel. Ten years following phenol peeling the patient shows the gravitational effects of aging, but there has been no recurrence of facial wrinkling. The longevity of phenol peeling is remarkable.

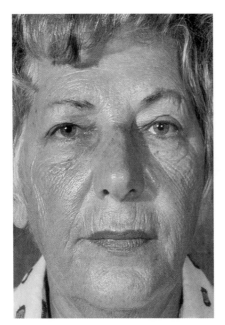 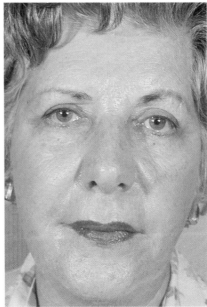

This patient sought treatment for coarse and fine facial rhytides. She had a face lift and subsequently a phenol peel. She is shown 6 months following chemical resurfacing.

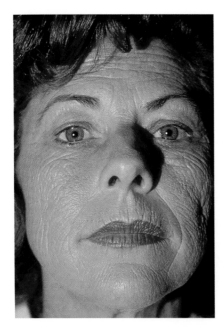 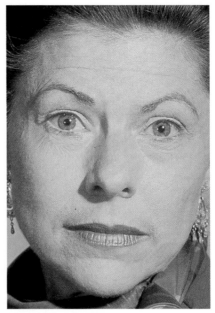

Six months following a full-face phenol peel this patient's coarse facial wrinkles have been totally eliminated. Observe the resulting hypopigmentation following full-face phenol application.

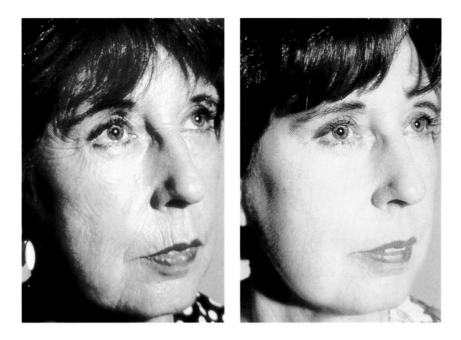

This 48-year-old patient exhibits severe photoaging. She is shown 1 year following a full-face phenol peel. No surgery was performed.

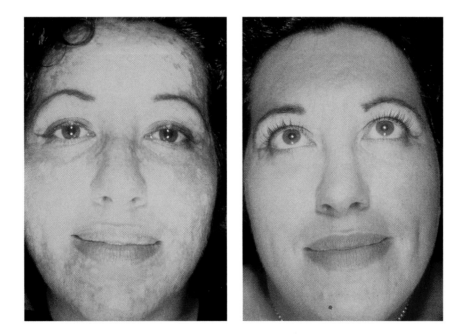

This patient complained of severe, blotchy hyperpigmentation that developed following a generalized allergic drug reaction. Seven months after a full-face phenol peel her complexion is uniform in color with no hyperpigmentation.

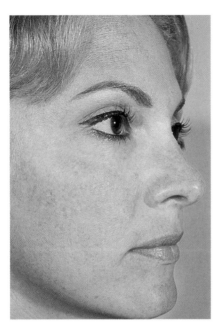 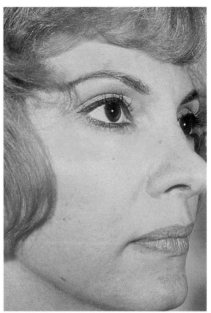

This patient's uniform hyperpigmentation was caused by prolonged exposure to sunlight. The blotchy pigmentation has not recurred 2 years after a full-face phenol peel. In retrospect, if we were treating this patient today, we most likely would have placed her on a skin care regimen followed by a medium-depth TCA peel rather than performing a deep phenol peel.

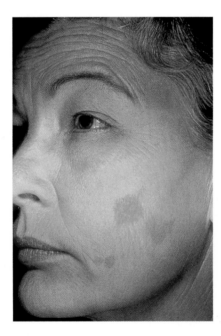 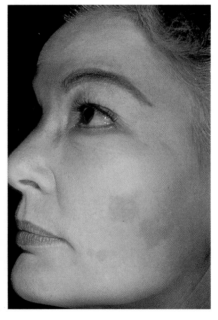

This patient has facial rhytides and port-wine stains of the cheek. She is shown following a full-face phenol peel. There is a significant improvement in facial wrinkling, but the port-wine stains have not diminished

COMPLICATIONS AND UNDESIRABLE RESULTS

When the phenol peel is performed as described, serious complications are rare. Some undesirable results, however, are to be expected, and these should be discussed with the patient.

Skin Depigmentation

Histologic examination of skin that has undergone phenol chemical peeling invariably demonstrates a reduction in the melanin-producing cells, thereby causing skin depigmentation. This bleaching effect is almost unavoidable except in the fairest of fair-skinned patients and is most noticeable at the line of demarcation just beneath the jawline. Individuals who have a confluence of freckles and other sun-induced blotches and individuals with red hair and ruddy complexions exhibit the most pronounced line of demarcation. We usually recommend another form of treatment for patients with this type of skin.

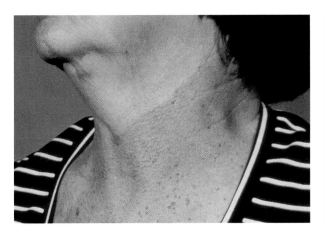 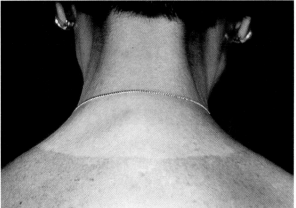

The importance of camouflaging the line of demarcation below the mandibular border is seen in these types of patients. In the patient on the left note that when the peel is carried more caudal on the neck the distinction between peeled and unpeeled skin is more obvious. Note also the scarring of the submental region following phenol application to cervical skin. We avoid the application of phenol to this region because of the lack of adnexal structures present within the neck. In this patient phenol application was carried to the base of the neck. In the patient on the right note the obvious line of demarcation when phenol peeling is performed in this location.

Erythema

The peeled area will become erythematous and appear quite red in the first few days following the peel. This erythema subsides gradually. After 12 to 14 days most patients can wear camouflaging makeup. However, in some patients this pinkness may persist for 10 to 12 weeks or even longer. In none of our patients has erythema been permanent. We treat patients with prolonged erythema with topical steroids, but to date we remain unconvinced of the efficacy of this treatment. Tincture of time combined with liberal doses of reassurance and support seems to be the best therapy.

Sensitivity to Sunlight

The skin will exhibit increased sensitivity to sunlight immediately after the chemical peel; this may persist for months. Consequently, all patients are instructed to use sunscreen daily for at least 4 to 6 months. Patients are also advised that their skin will never tan as it did before the procedure and they should continue to use a protective sunscreen on a daily basis.

Postpeel Hyperpigmentation

Postpeel hyperpigmentation is perhaps the most common problem seen following phenol peeling. It is most commonly noted in patients who have types III or IV skin or who have not protected themselves from sun exposure. It is imperative to stress to postpeel patients that while there is erythema they must avoid the sun, use sunscreens to block UVA rays, and wear opaque makeup to avoid the risk of hyperpigmentation. Should this troublesome complication develop, the pigmentation is usually limited to the superficial epidermis and dermis and is amenable to topical application of Retin-A, hydroquinone, and glycolic acids. These creams should be administered at the first sign of pigmentation. If pigmentation persists after several months on an adequate skin care regimen, medium-depth TCA peeling will usually be necessary.

Infection

Although an occasional case of superficial contamination of an open peeled area is encountered, none of our patients has developed true infection in the peeled areas. If these superficial areas appear to be inflamed or infected, they are treated with conventional antibiotics, both topical and parenteral.

We have seen more herpesvirus infections occur than when we first started performing phenol peels. If a patient has a history of perioral herpes simplex, the chances of developing a postpeel herpetic infection is approximately 50%. For this reason, any patient with a positive history of herpesvirus infections should be prophylactically treated with 400 mg acyclovir three times a day 24 hours prior to peeling and for 5 days after the peel. Alternatively, 500 mg of valacyclovir (Valtrex) twice a day can be used. If a herpes infection develops in a postpeel patient who has not had prophylactic therapy, 800 mg acyclovir three times a day is given and topical acyclovir ointment used until the infection resolves. Despite their clinical appearance, herpes infections are usually superficial lesions that respond to treatment rapidly and rarely result in residual scarring.

Milia

Milia occasionally occur after a phenol peel as a consequence of the healing process. These small, superficial inclusion cysts may appear at any time during the first few weeks after treatment. They are usually scattered but can be numerous and confluent. Most cases last a few days, but some can last several weeks. After the healing process is completed, frequent, vigorous washings and scrubbing later on will solve the problem. In rare cases of persistent milia it may be necessary to puncture the small milia under magnification in the office.

Scarring

Scarring is the rarest but most catastrophic complication of peeling. We have observed only rare instances of scarring with slight degrees of hypertrophy. This scarring has occurred in small areas on the upper lip, such as a transverse band of hypertrophic scar across the middle of the upper lip. These are generally minor and can be treated with intralesional steroids and topical steroids. They usually subside over a period of months; however, this problem is upsetting to the patient and to the treating physician alike. The worst scarring that we have seen has been on the anterior surface of the neck. Most of these patients were treated by lay operators. It has been our policy not to use phenol formula on the neck skin.

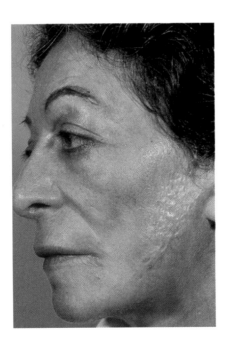

Hypertrophic scarring of the cheek developed in this patient following a phenol peel performed by a lay operator.

Ectropion of the Lower Eyelid

Early ectropion of the lower lid has been observed in some patients who have had a blepharoplasty. Usually this will subside spontaneously, although we have seen two cases in which a full-thickness skin graft or a canthopexy was required to correct this problem. An unrecognized incipient senile ectropion will contribute to this complication.

Alteration of Existing Skin Condition

Darkening of nevi is common after a phenol peel because the skin becomes lighter and the nevus becomes darker. If this skin condition is observed preoperatively, this potential problem should be discussed with the patient. Hyperkeratoses are usually completely removed by the peeling process, and on rare occasions we have advised patients to undergo the peeling procedure to remedy this problem. It has been observed that this reduces rather than increases the likelihood of the treated skin developing superficial malignancies. We have never seen skin cancer in a patient who has undergone a phenol peel. Patients who have spider telangiectasias should be told that the process will make these blood vessels more visible. If the telangiectatic areas are more visible after peeling, they can be treated appropriately. Some individuals request a peel to reduce the size of their pores. The peeling process generally leaves the pores unchanged. In fact, in some individuals it may make them appear somewhat larger.

CONCLUDING THOUGHTS

It is difficult to improve on the clinical results obtained with phenol peeling. The great limitation with this treatment agent is the frequent pigmentation and textural changes that occur following treatment. We find we use phenol peeling with less frequency and are relying more often on alternative agents such as dermabrasion and laser resurfacing. We still believe phenol is the most consistent agent available to obliterate coarse facial rhytides. Although other treatment agents are not as potent or as reliable as phenol, the reduced bleaching effect greatly broadens their applicability. The longevity of results following laser resurfacing has yet to be determined. Ultimately the use of phenol will largely depend on future research and clinical experience with laser resurfacing as well as the development of new treatment modalities.

REFERENCES

Baker TJ. The ablation of rhytides by chemical means: A preliminary report. J Fla Med Assoc 47:451, 1961.

Baker TJ. Chemical face peeling and rhytidectomy. A combined approach for face rejuvenation. Plast Reconstr Surg 29:199, 1962.

Baker TJ, Gordon HL. Chemical face peeling, an adjunct to surgical face lifting. South Med J 56:412, 1963.

Baker TJ, Gordon HL. Chemical face peeling and dermabrasion. Surg Clin North Am 51:387, 1971.

Baker TJ, Gordon HL. Chemical peeling as a practical method of removing rhytides of the upper lip. Ann Plast Surg 2:209, 1979.

Baker TJ, Gordon HL. Chemical face peeling. In Surgical Rejuvenation of the Face. St. Louis: CV Mosby, 1986.

Baker TJ, Stuzin JM. Chemical peeling and dermabrasion. In McCarthy JG, ed. Plastic Surgery. Philadelphia: WB Saunders, 1990, p 45.

Baker TJ, Gordon HL, Seckinger DL. A second look at chemical face peeling. Plast Reconstr Surg 37:487, 1966.

Baker TJ, Gordon HL, Stuzin JM. Chemical peeling (phenol and trichloroacetic acid) and dermabrasion. In Surgical Rejuvenation of the Face, 2nd ed. St. Louis: Mosby, 1996, p 45.

Baker TJ, Gordon HL, Mosienko P, Seckinger DL. Long-term histological study of skin after chemical face peeling. Plast Reconstr Surg 53:522, 1974.

Brown AM, Kaplan LM, Brown ME. Phenol-induced histological skin changes: Hazards, techniques, and uses. Br J Plast Surg 13:158, 1960.

Deichmann W, Witherup S. Phenol studies. VI. The acute and comparative toxicity of phenol and o-, m-, and p-cresols for experimental animals. J Pharmacol Exp Ther 80:233, 1944.

Gross BG. Cardiac arrhythmias during phenol face peeling. Plast Reconstr Surg 73:590, 1984.

Litton C. Chemical face lifting. Plast Reconstr Surg 29:371, 1962.

Litton C. Follow-up study of chemosurgery. South Med J 50:1007, 1966.

Stuzin JM, Baker TJ, Gordon HL. Treatment of photoaging: Facial chemical peeling (phenol and trichloroacetic acid) and dermabrasion. Clin Plast Surg 20:9, 1993.

Stuzin JM, Baker TJ, Gordon HL. Chemical peel—A change in routine. Ann Plast Surg 22:301, 1989.

Truppman ES, Ellenby JD. Major electrocardiographic changes during chemical face peeling. Plast Reconstr Surg 63:44, 1979.

7

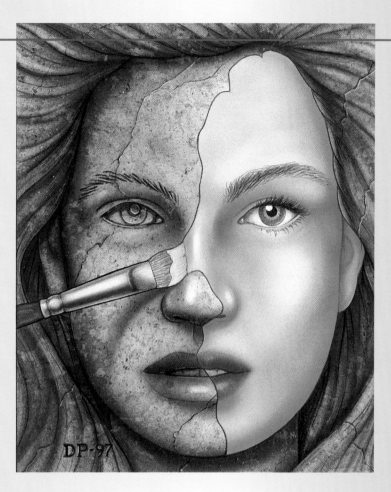

Dermabrasion

Although dermabrasion is a time-tested modality for the treatment of rhytides and acne scarring, in recent years this technique has been largely overshadowed by laser resurfacing. Dermabrasion, however, has much to recommend it. In the rush to embrace laser technology and accommodate public demand, we must not overlook the merits of dermabrasion while emphasizing its shortcomings. It is effective, convenient, and applicable to a broad spectrum of patients. Abundant clinical and histologic studies have confirmed its efficacy. The equipment required is inexpensive and portable. Because dermabrasion is associated with a shorter erythema phase than either phenol peeling or laser resurfacing, it may be particularly appealing to patients who ordinarily wear little or no makeup and wish to resume normal activities as soon as possible. The erythema after dermabrasion generally resolves in 4 to 6 weeks as compared with 8 to 12 weeks for laser therapy. Cost may also affect patient decision making. Because of the expense of the laser machine, the fees for dermabrasion tend to be lower.

Dermabrasion is not without shortcomings. The effectiveness of treatment is largely determined by the technical skill of the operator. Because of the variations in technique, undertreatment may lead to inadequate results and overtreatment may result in hypopigmentation or, in severe cases, scarring.

We commonly use dermabrasion as an adjunct for treating perioral rhytides in patients undergoing simultaneous surgical rejuvenation of the aging face. Compared with laser resurfacing, the equipment requirements for dermabrasion are simple and the success rate equivalent. Since dermabrasion requires no corneal protection or fire safety restrictions, patient safety is enhanced. Even if laser resurfacing is to be performed on other areas of the face (e.g., crow's-feet and glabella), the perioral region can be dermabraded with predictable improvement of coarse rhytides and more rapid resolution of posttreatment erythema.

MECHANISM OF ACTION

Dermabrasion is the controlled mechanical planing of the epidermis and a variable portion of the upper dermis using a rotating abrasive mechanical wheel to smooth rhytides and improve scars. The shoulders of rhytides can be *mechanically* lowered and smoothed. Similarly, the topographic irregularity of scars can be leveled, resulting in a more uniform contour of the skin surface. Dermabrasion predictably ameliorates coarse facial rhytides as the fibroplasia of wounding results in neocollagen formation along the upper level of the dermis. The wound produced heals by reepithelialization from the dermal appendages.

INDICATIONS AND PATIENT SELECTION

Dermabrasion is indicated for the treatment of perioral rhytides as well as acne and posttraumatic facial scarring. The upper lip is particularly amenable to treatment when the goal is ablation of "smoker's lines." Similar lines on the lower lip, however, are more intransigent and frequently persistent rhytides, especially along the vermilion border, will require secondary resurfacing. In addition, dermabrasion remains the standard treatment for rhinophyma.

The delicate upper and lower eyelid skin is too thin to tolerate mechanical abrasion, and other forms of resurfacing are more appropriate.

Rhinophyma

Dermabrasion remains a fundamental tool for the treatment of rhinophyma. This clinical condition is marked by severe hyperplasia of the sebaceous glands. Clinically, an insidious enlargement of the nose results in bulbous contours and interspersed nodules. The skin becomes hyperemic and congested. Microscopic examination reveals sebaceous gland hypertrophy or hyperplasia, dermal fibrovascular proliferation, and epithelial acanthosis. In more severe cases, surgical extirpation followed by dermabrasion for final contouring is the treatment of choice.

Scars

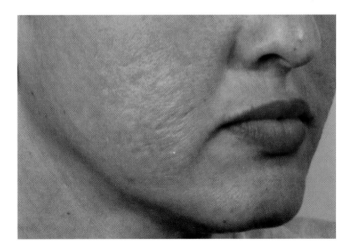

Acne scars typically present as depressed areas of varying diameter and depth. Small scars can be successfully treated with dermabrasion. Moderate and severe scars will show improvement but are rarely eliminated even with repeated treatments. Each resurfacing attempt will produce a 30% to 50% overall improvement in scar appearance.

Posttraumatic scars may be elevated or depressed and are approached in a similar fashion. The surface contour is evened out by mechanically sanding the elevated regions down to the level of the depressions. The results of laser resurfacing and dermabrasion appear to be similar in these patients.

Perioral Rhytides

Perioral rhytides can be treated using dermabrasion (mechanical), peeling (chemical), or laser (ablative vaporization) techniques. The method selected is influenced by the nature of the pathology, the skin type, and the surgeon's expertise and comfort level. Other considerations include technologic capabilities, patient desires, anticipated morbidity, and cost.

The severity of the pathology is perhaps the single most important factor in the selection process. Rhytides may arbitrarily be classified as mild, moderate, or severe based on depth and number.

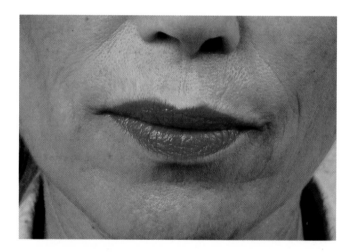

Type I rhytides are mild or superficial; they originate at the vermilion border and extend to an area covering no more than half of the upper lip. The number of rhytides is limited. The lower lip is less affected. These rhytides are the stigmata of early aging, accentuated by smoking and sun damage.

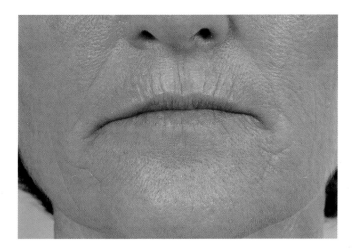

Type II rhytides are of moderate depth and extend to an area that covers up to two thirds of the upper lip. Lower lip involvement is common.

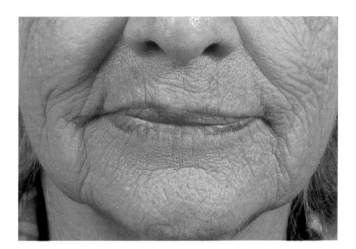

Type III rhytides are coarse and deep and involve the full extent of the upper lip. The lower lip and chin complex are similarly involved.

Dermabrasion is an effective modality for treating perioral rhytides. Patients with types I and II rhytides require lighter treatments and have a shorter duration of posttreatment erythema as compared with patients who have extensive coarse rhytides.

Skin type also affects treatment planning. Patients with Fitzpatrick types I to III skin, who exhibit mild to moderate rhytides, are ideal candidates for all resurfacing modalities. The pigment characteristics of patients with Fitzpatrick type IV skin are especially critical in selecting the proper technique. Regional phenol application is not appropriate in these types of patients. Dermabrasion is associated with less hypopigmentation than phenol, although long-term follow-up often reveals pigmentary changes in patients treated for coarse facial rhytides. Even laser resurfacing can produce troublesome bleaching if the level of resurfacing is deep, but it seems to be the best option in patients with type IV skin. There is no perfect treatment modality for deep facial wrinkling.

TECHNIQUE

We perform dermabrasion in an operating room setting after the patient is sedated and the skin infiltrated with local anesthetic solution.

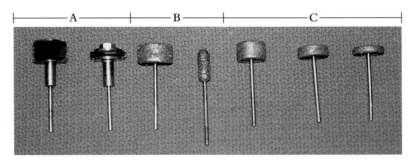

A, Wide and narrow wire brushes; **B,** wide and cylindric coarse fraises; **C,** wide, medium, and narrow fine fraises.

The hand-held dermabrader is an electrically powered, motor-driven unit with interchangeable heads. Wire brushes, sandpaper-covered cylinders, and stainless steel burrs are available. We prefer an assortment of diamond-impregnated cylindric fraises. They are available in a wide variety of shapes and sizes with variable coarseness. Gradual and controlled planing can be achieved by driving these fraises at 12,000 to 15,000 rpm. Fine rather than coarse fraises allow the procedure to proceed at a safer and more comfortable pace.

Care should be taken to protect the surgeon and operating room personnel from exposure to the aerosolized particulate matter dispersed during dermabrasion. Hepatitis and AIDS viruses are of particular concern. Appropriate gown, glove, mask, and eyewear protection are essential.

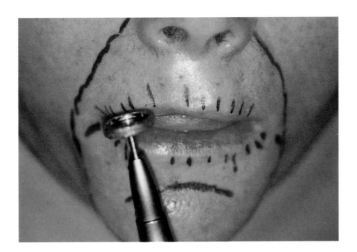

This patient has been marked for perioral dermabrasion following a face lift and lower lid blepharoplasty. Prior to the administration of the anesthetic the area to be treated is outlined with ink and the individual rhytides and transverse mental crease marked. Regions of treatment should correlate with anatomic subunits.

The skin is placed under gentle spreading tension using the thumb and index finger of the nondominant hand. The shape and size of the dermabrading fraise chosen will depend on the anatomic area to be treated and the surgeon's preference. We generally use a narrow 5 mm wheel-shaped head for abrasion along the vermilion border and a larger, broader cylindric fraise over flatter regions of the lip and cheek. The plane of the fraise should be kept parallel to the skin's surface and moved with light brushing strokes. Light pressure allows the motor to do the work and helps prevent heat buildup through friction. The handpiece is kept moving continuously during the procedure to disperse heat and maintain an even level of planing throughout the treated field. At the periphery the depth of the planing is decreased. Feathering along the edge helps blend the treated and untreated areas.

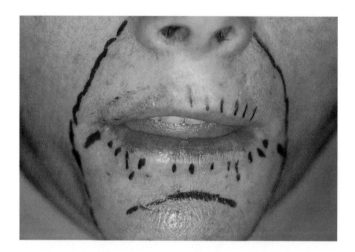

Determining the proper depth of wounding is critical. If the wound is too superficial, rhytides will remain; if too deep, hypertrophic scarring may result. As
the planing progresses, the outer tan-colored epithelium is removed, revealing
the pinker dermal–epidermal junction.

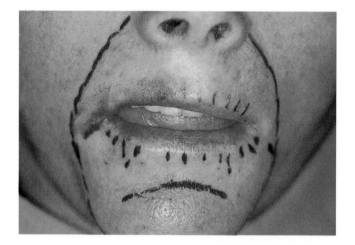

As the depth increases, sparse punctate bleeding points are seen on a smooth
pink background. This level represents the superficial papillary dermis.

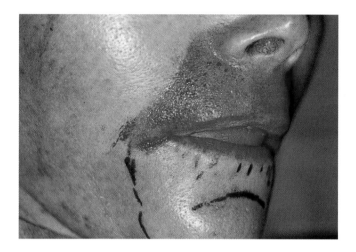

Bleeding points are more numerous as the depth of the abrasion increases, and the smooth pink background takes on a slightly rougher appearance. This corresponds to the deep papillary or papillary-reticular junction and represents the end point of treatment for most patients with mild to moderate rhytides. If planing is continued, the abraded area takes on a rough, irregular appearance as more of the dermal collagen is exposed and begins to shred. This level must be approached cautiously. It is advisable to limit the abrasion and consider a secondary procedure if rhytides persist postoperatively.

For the treatment of rhinophyma, surgical extirpation reduces the affected outer layers. In mild cases of rhinophyma the sebaceous hyperplasia may be removed by dermabrasion alone. Coarse wire brushes are used first, and finer fraises are used for the final contouring. In more advanced cases the nodules and thicker dermal hyperplasia should be debulked by making a tangential excision with the scalpel. Dermabrasion is then used to shape and detail the final contour. Because of the extensive network of epidermal appendages, contouring can be aggressive. Reepithelialization is usually complete within 7 to 10 days. Follow-up care is similar to that after dermabrasion of other areas of the face.

POSTTREATMENT CARE

A saline-moistened gauze sponge is placed over the abraded wound until hemostasis is achieved. A petrolatum-based ointment is then applied to the entire treated area and left uncovered. The patient is instructed to gently cleanse the region with tap water three or four times a day and reapply a light layer of the ointment. A & D ointment prevents the formation of eschar, keeps the wound lubricated, and allows the surgeon to easily check the progress of healing. Reepithelialization is complete within 7 to 10 days. The petrolatum ointment is discontinued after healing and a moisturizer is substituted.

Once reepithelialization has occurred, the healed region can be covered with makeup to help conceal the erythema, which gradually fades in 4 to 6 weeks. During this maturation phase and for several months thereafter the newly formed layers of skin are particularly sensitive to ultraviolet light. The physician should stress that the use of sunscreens is mandatory during this time. Postoperative treatment with Retin-A and hydroquinone will help prevent post-inflammatory pigmentation in patients with Fitzpatrick types III and IV skin.

RESULTS

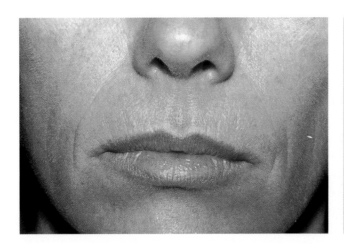 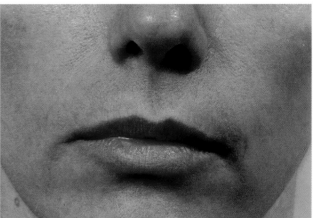

This patient had type I perioral rhytides. Mild hypopigmentation of the upper lip occurred after dermabrasion despite the superficial level of resurfacing.

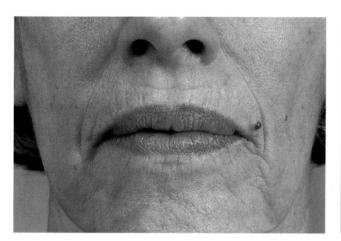 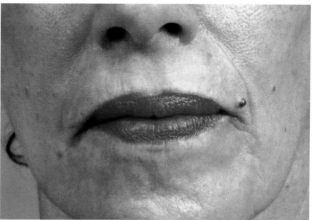

This patient with type II perioral rhytides underwent dermabrasion, but the lower lip rhytides did not respond to treatment. Persistent lower lip rhytides are common when treating this level of pathology, especially along the lower vermilion border. Hypopigmentation is evident along the upper lip.

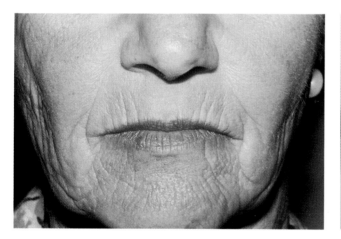 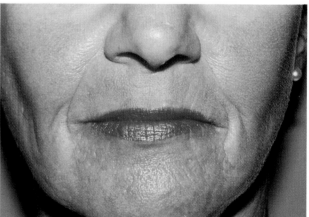

As demonstrated in this patient, dermabrasion produced significant improvement in perioral rhytides with minimal change in pigmentation. Pigmentary changes following dermabrasion are difficult to predict.

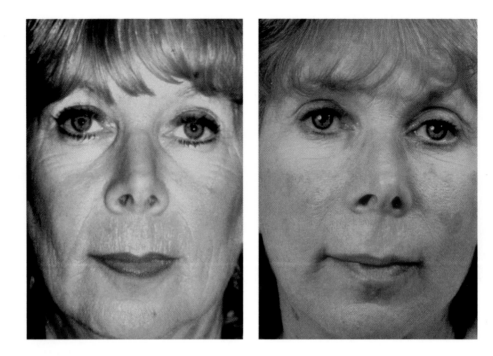

This patient with type II perioral rhytides is shown following rhytidectomy and dermabrasion.

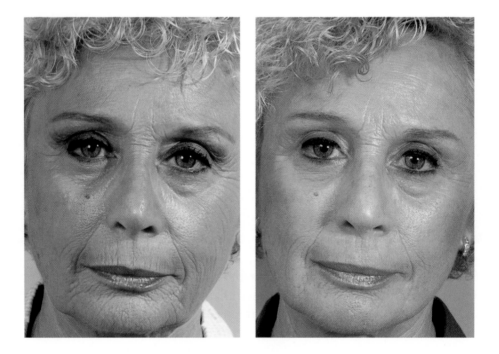

This woman exhibits early type III perioral rhytides. Note the complete involvement of the lower lip and chin pad. She is shown 1 year after a face lift and perioral dermabrasion. This patient had only a mild pigmentary change.

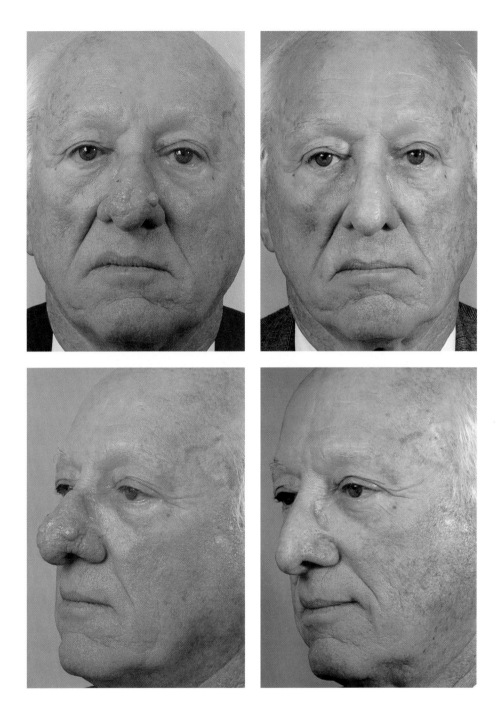

This man with moderate rhinophyma demonstrates the typical signs of sebaceous hyperplasia, nodules, and hypervascularity. He is shown 9 months after scalpel debulking and dermabrasion contouring.

COMPLICATIONS AND UNDESIRABLE RESULTS

The most feared complication of dermabrasion is hypertrophic scarring, which results from deep wounding or subsequent to infection. The key to prevention is recognition of the depth of abrasion.

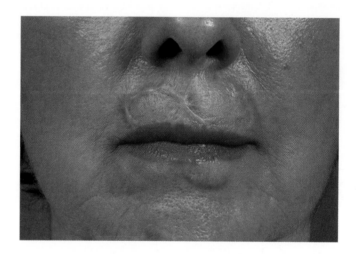

A herpes virus infection outbreak occurred in this patient who was not treated with prophylactic acyclovir. Hypotrophic scarring resulted. She was from out of town and left before healing was complete. She is seen 14 months following the initial procedure.

Signs of bacterial, fungal, or viral infection must be recognized early, cultures taken, and treatment started. Patients who have a history of perioral herpes simplex outbreaks should be given oral acyclovir or valacyclovir for prophylactic treatment. Signs of early hypertrophic scar formation mandate aggressive treatment. Wounds that take more than 14 days to heal should alert the physician to possible complications. Intralesional steroid injections, pressure garments, and silicone sheeting may be used for progressing or advanced hypertrophic scarring. Early, aggressive therapy is critical to prevent more serious, established scars.

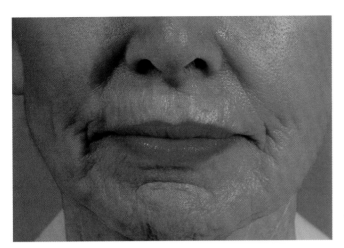 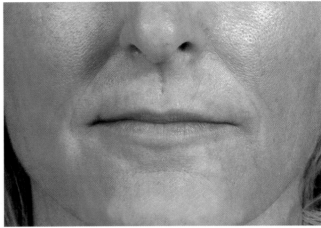

Hypopigmentation following dermabrasion occurs most frequently in patients with fair complexions who undergo aggressive resurfacing; however, alterations in color and texture may occur in any patient after dermabrasion. The patient on the left, who has Fitzpatrick type II skin, developed moderate hypopigmentation following dermabrasion for perioral rhytides. She is shown 9 years after treatment. Even though resurfacing was deep enough to alter pigmentation, several rhytides were not obliterated. The patient on the right, who also has Fitzpatrick type II skin, developed blotchy hypopigmentation of the upper and lower lip. She is shown 1 year after perioral resurfacing.

CONCLUDING THOUGHTS

Dermabrasion remains an important tool in our clinical practice despite its limitations. It is, in reality, a simple technique, and the key to consistency is patient selection and technical expertise. The predictability of dermabrasion for improving coarse rhytides must be weighed against the common occurrence of mild to moderate hypopigmentation. The "cold" injury of abrasion produces less posttreatment morbidity than laser resurfacing. The ability to lightly abrade some areas while specifically abrading the shoulders of coarse rhytides tends to promote more rapid healing. Overall, we remain impressed with the reliability of dermabrasion for treating perioral rhytides, scars, and rhinophyma even in the face of continued demand for laser resurfacing.

REFERENCES

Abadir DM, Abadir AR. Dermabrasion under regional anesthesia without refrigeration of the skin. J Dermatol Surg Oncol 6:119, 1980.

Alt TH. Therapeutic facial dermabrasion. In Epstein E, ed. Skin Surgery, 6th ed. Philadelphia: WB Saunders, 1987, p 327.

Baker TJ. The ablation of rhytides by chemical means: A preliminary report. J Fla Med Assoc 47:451, 1961.

Baker TJ. Chemical face peeling and rhytidectomy. A combined approach for face rejuvenation. Plast Reconstr Surg 29:199, 1962.

Baker TJ, Gordon HL. Chemical peeling and dermabrasion. Surg Clin North Am 51:387, 1971.

Baker TJ, Gordon HL. Chemical face peeling. In Baker TJ, Gordon HL, Stuzin JM. Rejuvenation of the Face. St. Louis: Mosby, 1986, p 37.

Baker TJ, Gordon HL, Stuzin JM. Ancillary procedures. In Surgical Rejuvenation of the Face, 2nd ed. St. Louis: Mosby, 1996, p 575.

Baker TJ, Stuzin JM. Chemical peeling and dermabrasion. In McCarthy JG, ed. Plastic Surgery, vol 3. Philadelphia: WB Saunders, 1990, p 748.

Baker TM, Stuzin JM, Baker TJ, Gordon HL. Adjunctive procedures to improve the facelift result: Chemical peels, dermabrasion, and autologous injection. In Grotting JC, ed. Reoperative Aesthetic and Reconstructive Plastic Surgery. St. Louis: Quality Medical Publishing, 1995, pp 295-321.

Baker TM, Stuzin JM, Baker TJ, Gordon HL. What's new in aesthetic surgery. Clin Plast Surg 23:3, 1996.

Barton FE Jr, Byrd HS. Acquired deformities of the nose. In McCarthy JG, ed. Plastic Surgery, vol 3. Philadelphia: WB Saunders, 1990, p 1987.

Behin F, Feuerstein SS, Marovitz W. Comparative histological study of mini pig skin after chemical peel and dermabrasion. Arch Otolaryngol 103:271, 1977.

Converse JM, Robb-Smith AHT. The healing of surface cutaneous wounds: Its analogy with the healing of superficial burns. Ann Surg 120:873, 1944.

Hill TG. Cutaneous wound healing following dermabrasion. J Dermatol Surg Oncol 6:487, 1980.

Kligman AM, Baker TJ, Gordon HL. Long-term histologic follow-up of phenol peels. Plast Reconstr Surg 75:652, 1985.

Kurtin A. Corrective surgical planing of skin: New technique for treatment of acne scars and other skin defects. Arch Dermatol Syph 68:389, 1953.

Orentreich N, Dunn NP. Dermabrasion. In Goldwyn RM, ed. The Unfavorable Result in Plastic Surgery, 2nd ed. Boston: Little, Brown, 1984, p 919.

Rees TD. Chemabrasion and dermabrasion. In Rees TD, ed. Aesthetic Plastic Surgery. Philadelphia: WB Saunders, 1980, p 749.

Ship AG, Weiss PR. Pigmentation after dermabrasion: An avoidable complication. Plast Reconstr Surg 75:528, 1985.

Stegman SJ. A study of dermabrasion and chemical peels in an animal model. J Dermatol Surg Oncol 6:490, 1980.

Stegman SJ. A comparative histologic study of the effects of three peeling agents and dermabrasion on normal and sun-damaged skin. Aesthetic Plast Surg 6:123, 1982.

Stuzin JM, Baker TJ, Gordon HL. Treatment of photoaging: Facial chemical peeling (phenol and trichloroacetic acid) and dermabrasion. Clin Plast Surg 20:18, 1993.

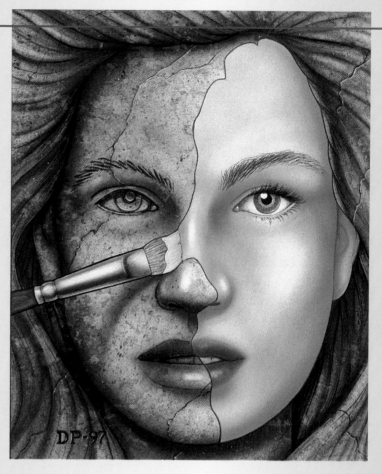

Fundamentals of Laser Surgery

The high-energy pulsed CO_2 laser has revolutionized the treatment of photoaged skin. The significance of this modality parallels the clinical investigation of phenol in the 1960s. Although newer, more precise lasers continue to be developed, the fundamental principles of laser surgery apply to all the instruments available and must be mastered by any physician who uses this modality for skin resurfacing.

Any new technology or treatment method involves a learning curve. Certainly laser resurfacing is no exception. The key to consistency and safety is learning the fundamentals of laser physics, the basic principles of laser resurfacing, and the safety measures that must be strictly followed by both physician and staff. Laser resurfacing is much more complex than simply setting a machine at a particular energy level and delivering a specific number of passes to actinically damaged skin. The physician must understand the interaction between the laser and the resurfaced tissue to ensure that the energy delivered to sun-damaged skin is appropriate for a particular patient. Adjustment in laser settings can have profound clinical ramifications that spell success or disaster. Only by gaining a thorough understanding of laser physics and safety can results be obtained that parallel those of chemical peeling or dermabrasion.

Albert Einstein first described the underlying principle of the laser in 1917. It would take nearly four decades for his theory to become a reality with the introduction of the first machines capable of producing laser light (stimulated emission). The first application of stimulated emission of radiation involved the microwave region of the electromagnetic spectrum (MASER). In 1958 Townes and Schawlow proposed extending the principles of MASER technology to devices that were designed to operate in the infrared and visible range of light. In 1960 Maiman stimulated a ruby crystal to produce a red laser light at a wavelength of $0.69~\mu$m. In 1961 the first lasers for medical use were developed using this ruby-stimulated crystal for ophthalmologic surgery. By 1966 neurosurgical resection of glioblastomas was reported. Further medical research led to the discovery of the continuous-wave CO_2 laser, which was developed for neurosurgery because of the need for high-power delivery to surgically resected tissue. With the CO_2 laser (the energy of which is absorbed by water), it was noted that thermal destruction to the surrounding tissue was limited and the depth of penetration was minimal. These qualities produced better hemostasis during tissue resection. Further technologic innovations using the YAG and argon lasers extended the use of laser technology to other medical specialities, including otolaryngology, dermatology, and plastic surgery. Further research and technologic improvements have given us a variety of lasers that offer greater precision and efficiency.

LASER PHYSICS

Laser is an acronym for *l*ight *a*mplification by *s*timulated *e*mission of *r*adiation. The principle is based on the theory that atoms are composed of a positively charged nucleus orbited by negatively charged electrons.

Atoms at Rest

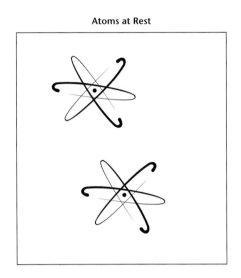

Spontaneous Emission

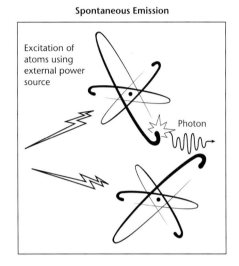

Excitation of atoms using external power source

Photon

Stimulated Emission

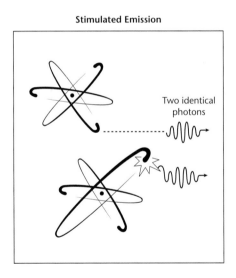

Two identical photons

Return to Normal State

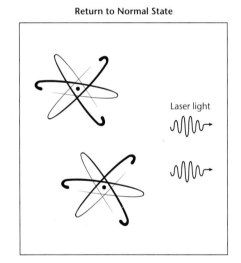

Laser light

When an atom is energized, electrons shift their orbits to a higher and less stable level. This is referred to as an *excited state*. Atoms in excited states seek to regain stability by dropping these electrons into lower orbits and emitting this energy as a *photon*. This series of events is termed *spontaneous emission of radiation*. These emitted photons will produce additional photons from similar atoms or molecules in excited states and will tend to travel in the same direction. Einstein termed these events *stimulated emission of radiation*.

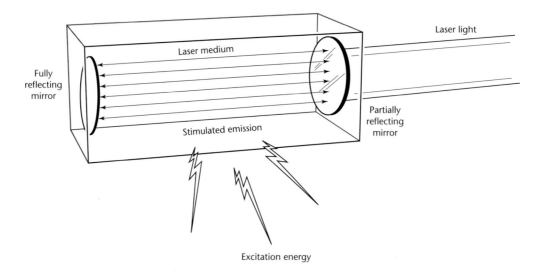

Many different substances are capable of producing laser light. These may take solid forms such as crystals, liquid dyes, or more commonly, mixtures of gases. Typically a gas mixture is placed into a cylindric container with a partially reflecting mirror at one end and a fully reflecting mirror at the other. When an external energy source is applied to this gas mixture, it produces many atoms in excited states. This is known as a *population inversion*. As these photons travel back and forth in this reflecting tube, they collide with other atoms in excited states to produce stimulated emission, a continuous stream of like photons. The partially reflecting mirror at one end of the laser allows a small fraction of this light to escape and produce the laser beam. This beam is then transmitted through the articulated arm via a series of precisely aligned mirrors and lenses to the working handpiece, which can then further focus and intensify the laser light.

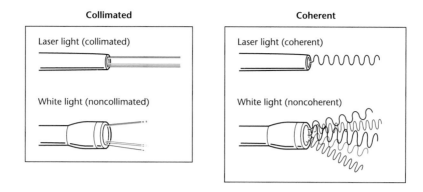

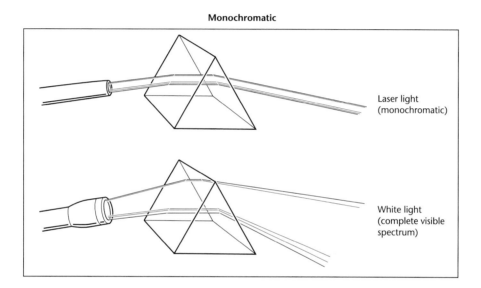

Lasers produce extraordinarily intense light beams that may be described as collimated, coherent, and monochromatic in contrast to ordinary white light. The *collimated* light produced by a laser travels over long distances in a single direction with little or no divergence of the beam. This produces extremely small spot sizes that enhance precision. Normal white light is a disorganized mixture of photons possessing many different directions, wavelengths, and phases. *Coherent* light moves in phase in time and space. That is, the peaks and troughs of the waves are aligned. Since photons travel at the speed of light and can be thought of as possessing wave characteristics under most circumstances, the wavelength is the distance between two peaks of consecutive waves. Thus, in wave theory, laser light is *monochromatic,* that is, all photons are of the same wavelength. This produces pure beams.

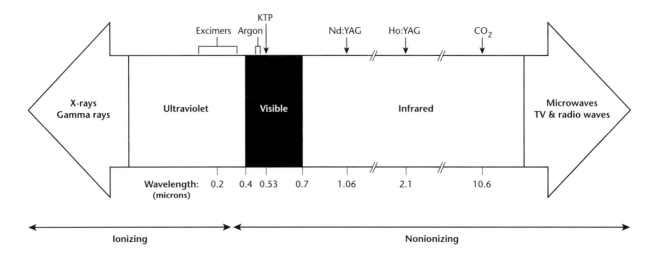

The compound(s) within the laser determines the wavelength. The electromagnetic spectrum organizes these wavelengths by size. Visible light ranges from 0.4 to 0.7 μm and represents the center of the electromagnetic spectrum. To the left are the shorter wavelengths of the ultraviolet spectrum, x-rays and gamma rays. To the right is the infrared spectrum and the longest wavelengths of microwaves and radio waves. Medical lasers representing the entire range of the electromagnetic spectrum are available. The most common include the CO_2, holmium:YAG, neodymium:YAG, argon ion, krypton ion, and helium-neon.

PROPERTIES OF SURGICAL LASERS*†

Laser Type	Laser Wavelength (nm)	Active Medium	Excitation Source	Power Range (watt)	Absorbing Chromosome	Absorbing Length (mm)
CO_2	10600	CO_2, N_2, He gas mixture	DC discharge or RF discharge	<1 to >100	Water	0.02
Ho:YAG	2140	Holmium in yttrium-aluminum-garnet	Flashlamp	<1 to 20	Water	0.5
Nd:YAG	1064	Neodymium in yttrium-aluminum-garnet	Flashlamp	<1 to >100	Dark-colored tissue	3–4
HeNe	633	Helium-neon	DC discharge	0.001 to 0.025	Dark-colored tissue	2–3
Dye	400–800	Organic compound in solution	Argon or krypton lasers; flashlamps	<1 to 5	Pigmented lesions	2–3
Frequency-doubled Nd:YAG (KTP)	532	Neodymium in yttrium-aluminum-garnet	Flashlamp	<1 to 20	Hemoglobin, melanin	2–3
Argon	514	Argon ions	DC discharge	<1 to 15	Hemoglobin	1–2
	488	Argon ions	DC discharge			0.5–0.8
Excimers						
XeF	351	Xenon fluoride			Proteins and water	0.2
XeCl	308	Xenon chloride	DC discharge	<1 to 20		0.1
KrF	248	Krypton fluoride				<0.1
ArF	193	Argon fluoride				<0.1

*From Trost D, Zacherl A, Smith MFW. Surgical laser properties and their tissue interaction. In Smith MFW, McEneen JT Jr, eds. Neurological Surgery of the Ear. St. Louis: Mosby, 1992.

†Surgical lasers have been developed operating over an extraordinarily wide band of the electromagnetic spectrum ranging from mid-infrared to ultraviolet. In general the visible wavelengths have proved most effective in ophthalmology, whereas the infrared wavelengths are most effective in surgery outside the eye. The ultraviolet lasers remain largely experimental.

The CO_2 laser is the most widely used and versatile laser in medicine. It has a wavelength of 10.6 μm (20 times longer than visible light) and resides in the mid-infrared portion of the electromagnetic spectrum. This wavelength makes the beam of the CO_2 laser invisible. The gas within the laser tube is actually a mixture of CO_2, helium, and nitrogen. The external power source is typically radio frequency. Because of its invisible beam, the CO_2 laser is commonly coupled with a second laser that possesses a beam in the visible spectrum. The helium-neon laser is ideal for this application because it does not interact with tissue. Precise alignment of the CO_2 and helium-neon beams allows accurate aiming of the CO_2 laser.

LASER TERMINOLOGY

When the light beam is generated by the laser, it is passed through a series of mirrors and articulating arms to a handpiece, where it is focused and the energy concentrated. To help categorize the physical characteristics of the laser and its ability to standardize energy delivery to human skin, the following terminology has been developed.

energy   The capacity to do work measured in joules. It is calculated in laser surgery as power multiplied by time of application and essentially represents a dosage measurement.

power   Measurement of performance of work or the flow of energy. Mathematically, power is calculated by the energy delivered divided by the time of application. The unit of measurement of power is watts (1 watt = 1 J/sec).

power density (irradiance)   The rate at which energy is delivered per unit area measured in watts per square centimeter. Mathematically, it is calculated as power divided by the surface area of the beam or spot size. A reduction in spot size will generally produce a fourfold increase of energy at the impact site. Power density is the principal determinant of the rate at which tissue is vaporized. High-power densities vaporize tissue more rapidly and completely.

fluence   Total laser energy delivered per unit area expressed as joules per square centimeter. Fluence is a product of power density and exposure time. Whereas power density determines the rate at which tissue is vaporized, the volume of tissue removed is a function of the amount of energy applied.

spot size   Controlled by the focusing lens or in noncollimated handpieces by moving the laser handpiece either away from or toward the target site. With noncollimated beams, a small variation in distance from the handpiece to the target can produce dramatic alterations in the diameter of the spot size, consequently affecting power density. A larger spot size requires higher power to compensate for dilution in power density.

pulse energy   The energy of one pulse of a pulsed laser is measured in millijoules. Continuous-beam CO_2 lasers can be delivered in short pulses known as superpulsing or ultrapulsing to deliver very short energy pulses at high peak powers. Q-switching is another method to pulse the laser, employing rotating mirrors, resulting in an accumulation of laser energy that produces a giant pulse of high power and extremely short duration.

thermal relaxation time   The time required for the lased tissue to lose 50% of heat through diffusion. Significant thermal diffusion will not occur if the pulse duration is shorter than the time it takes the heated layer to cool. This discovery has led to the development of pulsed lasers. These types of lasers deliver high bursts of laser for short durations that limit thermal injury. Resurfacing occurs through vaporization of tissue resulting from optical penetration, minimizing associated thermal injury. A pulse width of less than 950 μsec is short enough to prevent clinically significant thermal damage, forming the theoretic basis for the high-energy pulsed CO_2 laser.

CO_2 LASER/TISSUE INTERACTION

When a laser beam strikes tissue, four events can occur: absorption, reflection, scattering, and transmission. Absorption is the event primarily responsible for laser resurfacing. The tissue becomes rapidly heated, resulting in vaporization and coagulation. Reflection represents a negligible portion of the laser/tissue interaction but becomes a safety issue for the patient, physician, and operating room personnel and dictates the use of reflective eyewear. Scattering is the small portion of the laser beam whose direction is changed as it passes through tissue. These scattered photons generally pass on to be absorbed. There is no significant transmission with the CO_2 laser because of its high affinity for water and its shallow penetration depth.

Absorption length is defined by the depth to which the laser light must penetrate to be 63% absorbed. *Extinction length* is the depth the laser must penetrate before only 10% of the entering light remains. These terms help define the strength of absorption of a particular material or tissue at a given wavelength. Histologic studies confirm that tissue damage is minimal between one absorption length and one extinction length. These lengths will vary widely depending on the wavelength of the particular laser. As an example, the absorption length of the CO_2 laser in water is 20 μm compared to those in the visible spectrum, such as argon, whose absorption length can be over 100 meters.

The body is roughly 70% water and represents the perfect absorption medium for the CO_2 laser. The beam passes into the tissue and the majority of energy is absorbed by the intracellular water. This produces rapid intracellular heating, transforming the target tissue into a vapor plume. This vaporization carries a majority of heat away in the plume, minimizing conduction to adjacent tissue. Some heat is conducted away from the target site; this process has been termed *thermal relaxation*. As defined above, depth of penetration is a function of the wavelength of the laser and defines the absorption length (or minimum zone of damage). This distance is 0.02 mm for the CO_2 laser. The absorption length and thermal relaxation time together define a critical power density. This is the minimum power density required to avoid charring and limit thermal damage to a depth equal to one absorption length. For the CO_2 laser, this is 50 watts/mm². Stated simply, heat retained by the tissues must be conducted away faster than it is absorbed to avoid thermal buildup and damage to tissue beyond the target area.

Ablation performed at settings less than the critical power density may result in heat buildup, carbonization of tissue, and formation of char. At lower power settings less laser energy is carried off as plume vapor and more is retained as heat. This is a critical concept to understand since it seems to go against the physician's instinct. Turning the power to a lower setting in an attempt to increase the level of safety may produce the opposite effect, especially as more passes will be required for the desired clinical effect. *We generally prefer to resurface at high-energy levels and minimize the number of passes.* The desired clinical effect results from vaporization of tissue through optical penetration rather than conductive thermal injury.

This concept is of top priority in resurfacing (ablation) and has led to the development of pulsed lasers. The laser is designed to deliver its energy in "pulses"—short bursts of energy followed by longer periods when energy is not delivered. This allows the laser to be applied to the tissue in short pulses of extremely high energy with intervals between pulses that permit conducted heat to dissipate (thermal relaxation). The UltraPulse CO_2 laser by Coherent produces a 314 μsec pulse followed by a 39,686 μsec off period. This high-energy pulse is well above the minimum power density required for ablation and the pulse duration is shorter than the thermal relaxation time, thus allowing the tissue to cool completely before being subjected to the next laser pulse. With appropriate settings and proper technique, the majority of the laser energy is carried away as a vapor plume and little heat is allowed to build up in the adjacent tissues. This selective photothermolysis targets the epidermis and upper dermis, ablating pathology and stimulating neocollagen formation.

Depth of Penetration Per Pass

Understanding the depth of penetration per pass of the pulsed laser is the key to safety and consistency in resurfacing. Multiple passes (at least two) are required to obtain long-term improvement in photoaged skin. The epidermis is vaporized by the first pass. Subsequent passes penetrate into the dermis (papillary and upper reticular), vaporizing elastotic tissue and stimulating fibroplasia and neocollagen formation. The heat delivered by the CO_2 laser is also theorized to produce structural contracture of dermal collagen, which is clinically observed during the second or third pass. The long-term clinical effect of heat-induced collagen shrinkage is undetermined.

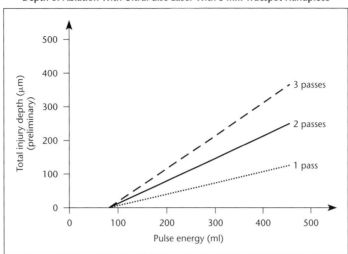

Depth of Ablation With UltraPulse Laser With 3 mm Truespot Handpiece

The depth of penetration per pass will depend on the type of laser used as well as the fluence delivered by the particular laser. Fitzpatrick observed that three passes of the Coherent UltraPulse laser produced an injury similar to dermabrasion (200 to 300 μm), only one fourth as deep as the injury produced by an application of Baker-Gordon phenol solution. In a more recent study Fitzpatrick found that the depth of penetration gradually leveled off, with penetration into the dermis decreasing with each subsequent pass. Specifically, he noted little increase in dermal penetration after the fourth pass. The level of penetration at four passes was approximately 250 mJ with 500 mJ of pulse energy. The residual thermal damage was approximately 100 μm, and this depth did not significantly increase even after 10 passes. Fitzpatrick concluded that single pulsed vaporization using the Coherent laser has a built-in safety mechanism whereby the depth of penetration is limited despite a large number of passes (as long as only single pulses are delivered without stacking).

Studies performed on human skin comparing the Sharplan and Coherent UltraPulse laser show approximately 20 to 40 μm of vaporization per pass, although the conductive thermal injury with the Sharplan SilkTouch scanner is twice as great as with the Coherent scanner; however, with the new Feather-Touch mode, the thermal injury is more comparable to that produced by the Coherent scanner. Whether these two laser systems produce significantly different clinical effects remains to be determined.

In clinical terms, it may be helpful to think of the first pass as vaporizing the epidermis and extending into the papillary dermis. The second pass ablates the papillary dermis and penetrates into the upper reticular dermis (this is our most common clinical depth of resurfacing). The third pass extends the penetration into the reticular dermis. Little penetration occurs after four passes, which explains why residual rhytides may be apparent despite aggressive laser resurfacing using multiple passes. Obviously the depth of penetration will vary from patient to patient depending on skin thickness and site being resurfaced. Also, the effects of stacking laser pulses (increasing spot size overlap or density) can increase thermal conduction and thus increase the depth of laser injury.

DETERMINING LASER DOSAGE

The laser settings for treating specific problems need to be determined preoperatively. Generally patients with thick, coarse rhytides require a greater degree of laser penetration and more tissue ablation to obtain the desired clinical effect. Patients with oily, acne-type skin have a greater margin of safety in terms of skin thickness and the ability to epithelialize deeper levels of resurfacing. When laser resurfacing is considered in patients with fine facial rhytides or pigmentation problems, lower energy settings can be used since tissue ablation does not need to be as deep. In general, when resurfacing at lower energy settings, less penetration is necessary, which means there is a shorter postoperative recovery. Specifically, postoperative erythema is minimized. On the other hand, when treating coarse facial rhytides, the axiom "no erythema, no long-term result" is often true. Depth of penetration is correlated with length of postoperative erythema, and in our practice the greatest improvement of coarse facial rhytides has been associated with a significant period of postoperative erythema.

Different areas of the face tolerate laser resurfacing differently. Delayed healing or scarring in the forehead or glabella is unusual. This region appears to tolerate laser resurfacing quite well despite multiple passes at high-energy levels. On the other hand, the eyelids have the thinnest of facial skin, and it is rare that more than two passes over the lower eyelids are required. The most difficult area to resurface is the perioral region. Perioral rhytides tend to be the deepest facial skin rhytides and the most recalcitrant to treatment. More than two passes are usually required to improve the perioral area; deep rhytides will remain even after four passes.

The key to depth of penetration is reading color change. If the skin following resurfacing turns to a tan chamois color, resurfacing should be terminated even if residual rhytides are still visible. Recalcitrant rhytides can be treated with a secondary procedure.

Suggested Parameters When Using the Coherent UltraPulse Computerized Programmed Generator (CPG) Scanner to Treat Different Areas of the Face

Perioral region
> Millijoules per pulse: 300
> Density: 5 to 6
> Number of passes: 2 to 4

Eyelids
> Millijoules: 300
> Density: 5 to 6
> Number of passes: 1 pass at 300 mJ and 1 pass at 150 mJ

Lateral canthus (crow's-feet)
> Millijoules: 300
> Density: 5 to 6
> Number of passes: 2 to 3

Upper eyelids
> Millijoules: 300
> Density: 5 to 6
> Number of passes: 1

Forehead and cheeks
> Millijoules: 300
> Density: 5 to 6
> Number of passes: 2 to 4

Nose
> Millijoules: 300
> Density: 5 to 6
> Number of passes: 1 to 2

NOTE: The thickness of the patient's skin, the type of pathology being treated, and color changes occurring with each pass must also be factored into the equation.

CASE EXAMPLES

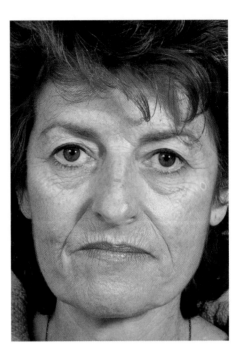

This patient exhibits fine rhytides of the lower eyelids, crow's-feet, and glabella. Coarser rhytides are seen on her upper lip and lower vermilion border. The rest of her face is fair and unlined. If full-face laser resurfacing is to be performed in a patient such as this, treatment should be concentrated on the lower eyelids, crow's-feet, and perioral regions. We would resurface the lower eyelids using the CPG scanner set at 300 mJ and a density of 5; for the crow's-feet we would use 300 mJ at a density of 6. Her perioral rhytides will prove challenging. We would first take down the shoulders of the rhytides using the 3 mm handpiece at 500 mJ. Following this, we would resurface the upper lip and lower vermilion border using two passes of the CPG scanner set at 300 mJ and a density of 6. A third pass might prove necessary depending on color changes. We would resurface the cheeks and forehead with the CPG scanner set at 300 mJ and a density of 5.

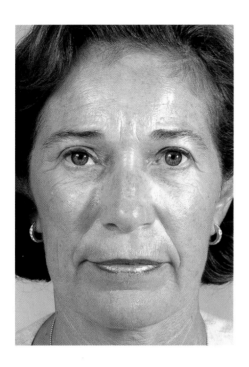

Chronic sun exposure in this patient has resulted in blotchy hyperpigmentation. A daily skin care program or medium-depth TCA peel is an option in this case. If resurfacing with the CO_2 laser is planned, pretreatment with Retin-A and hydroquinone is important to prevent postinflammatory pigmentation. Two passes over her entire face with the CPG scanner set at 300 mJ and a density of 5 are indicated. At least two passes at a density of 6 to treat upper lip rhytides would be needed.

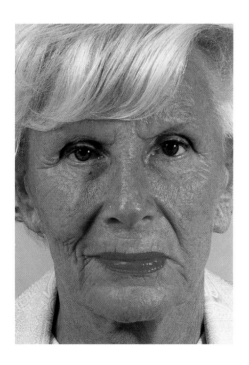

This patient shows signs of prolonged photodamage that has produced both coarse and fine facial rhytides and mottled pigmentation. We would use at least two passes of the CPG scanner set at 300 mJ and a density of 6. This would be the minimum treatment required to improve her coarse facial rhytides. The crow's-feet, perioral area, forehead, and glabella would require an extra one to two passes at this same density to remove the coarse rhytides in these areas.

TYPES OF LASERS

The two most commonly used CO_2 laser systems for resurfacing in the United States today are from Coherent and Sharplan. Although the physics is the same for both of these laser systems, there are some notable differences.

Coherent

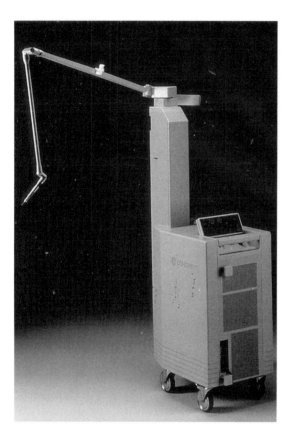
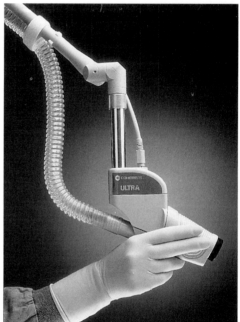

The UltraPulse 5000 series coupled with a CPG scanner is the laser we use in our office. The CPG scanner is a computer-driven control system that offers precision and accuracy. The handpiece is somewhat bulky but greatly reduces resurfacing times. The CPG scanner can be used to resurface large areas of precisely placed grids, up to 2 cm in size. The computer can be controlled to change the shape, size, or density (overlap) of these grids. Although each individual 2.2 mm collimated laser spot within the grid may be controlled as needed, the scanner is routinely set at 300 mJ. Adjusting the power (watts) will determine how quickly each grid is laid down.

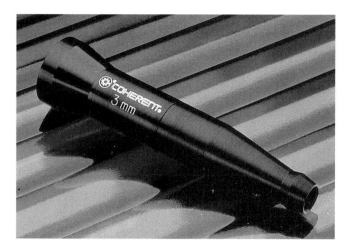

For very fine work, a 3 mm Truespot handpiece that generates a single 3 mm collimated spot may be used. Both of the handpieces produce collimated beams so there is no mandatory working distance.

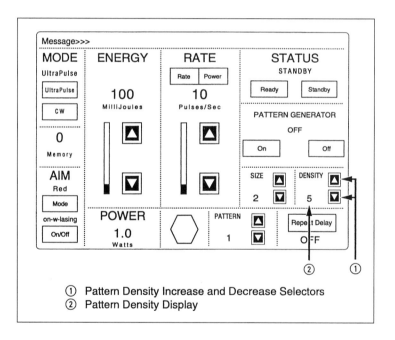

The display on the Coherent machine is large and easy to read. Settings include energy in millijoules that determines laser intensity, power in watts that reflects working speed, and several options to customize your routine. Note the fluence of this laser is 5 J/cm². The helium–neon beam intensity can be adjusted or set to "off while lasing." The laser is activated by depressing a footswitch. In the CPG mode this triggers the computer to produce a single preselected pattern. Alternatively, the footswitch can be set to repeat the pattern at a predicted time interval.

The CPG scanner has a series of pattern numbers that increase pattern size. The most common pattern used in our office is the number 3 pattern, which is a rectangular pattern. Smaller size patterns are useful for working along the lower eyelid and vermilion border. When large areas such as the forehead or cheek are being treated, the largest pattern available is used so that the resurfacing can be performed in a rapid fashion.

Pattern Density Number	1	2	3	4	5	6	7	8	9
Pattern Density Percentage	-10%	0%	10%	20%	30%	35%	40%	50%	60%
Available Pattern Sizes	1-5	1-6	1-7	1-8	1-9	1-9	1-9	1-9	1-9

The pattern density setting is more important than the pattern size. Pattern density adjusts spot size overlap, which affects the energy delivery and depth of penetration. The most common pattern density numbers that we use are density numbers 5 and 6. These correspond to a 30% to 35% spot size overlap. When working with coarse facial rhytides, we occasionally use a density of 7, which correlates with a 40% spot size overlap. Working at high-pulse energies and medium- to high-density levels increases the degree of tissue ablation through optical penetration while minimizing the underlying conductive thermal damage. It is always preferable to reach the desired depth of penetration with fewer passes, thereby ensuring tissue ablation through vaporization rather than conducted thermal injury.

Sharplan

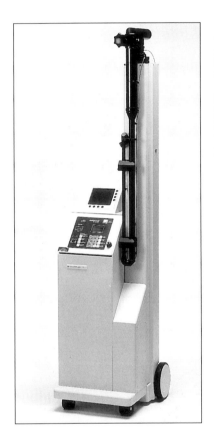

Char-free Vaporization Using the Dual-Mode Scanner

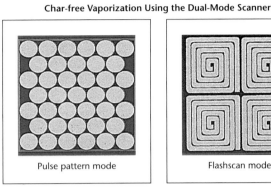

Pulse pattern mode

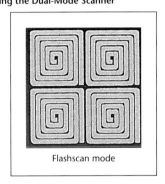

Flashscan mode

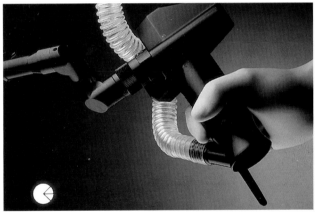

Sharplan produces the XJ dual-mode laser system with FeatherTouch flashscan technology as well as a new truly pulsed laser that is attached to a collimated computerized handpiece similar to the Coherent models. The FeatherTouch is not actually a pulsed laser but employs a focused continuous-wave CO_2 laser beam rapidly scanned circular or spiral pattern on the skin. The laser in either FeatherTouch mode or high-energy pulse mode is in contact with any single region of the skin surface for only a short time (less than 1 msec). The critical parameter of energy density is clearly displayed in joules/cm² on the laser screen.

The FeatherTouch flashscan technology vaporizes a volume of tissue in one pass and can be easily adjusted by increasing the laser power to treat superficial or deep pathology. This mode uses a focused handpiece with a guide tip to indicate the working distance that optimizes homogeneous vaporization. Angling or defocusing the handpiece allows for feathering to eliminate a sharp line of demarcation between treated and untreated areas.

The second mode of this dual-mode scanner is similar to the Coherent Ultra-Pulse. The high-energy pulse pattern generator provides tissue vaporization with minimal thermal damage. Employing a preprogrammed scan pattern with adjustable density, the pulse pattern mode allows precise control of tissue effect for the desired depth of vaporization and collagen shrinkage level.

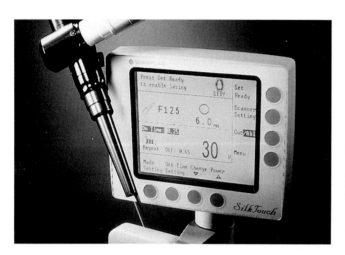 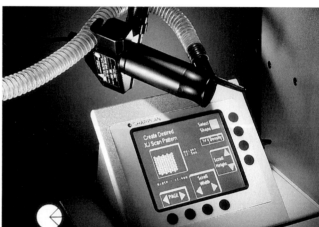

Additionally, Sharplan produces smaller, more compact, and less expensive CO_2 lasers that incorporate the FeatherTouch and SilkTouch flashscan technology. The difference between the two modes is in the pulse width or dwell time. The FeatherTouch, as mentioned, can treat superficial or deep pathology with minimal residual thermal injury. The SilkTouch is most effective for treating significant photoaging and acne scarring and is generally associated with more prolonged posttreatment erythema than the FeatherTouch. This mode again uses a focused handpiece to effectively vaporize tissue and a defocused beam to blend areas of the face. Whether using a collimated or focused handpiece it is imperative to stay close to tissue in following the curves and planes of the face.

Pulsed Erbium/YAG Laser

The Er/YAG laser is currently being studied for dermatologic applications. This laser appears to have a greater specificity for tissue interaction than the CO_2 laser at similar fluence levels. At low fluences the Er/YAG laser can ablate between 10 and 30 μm of tissue per pass as opposed to the CO_2 laser, which can ablate approximately 50 to 100 μm of tissue per pass. Two to three passes with the Er/YAG laser are sufficient to remove the epidermis with minimal adjacent char. Because of the low depth of penetration per pass, this laser can be selectively used to treat superficial epidermal and dermal pathology. Preliminary reports indicate that posttreatment erythema persists for less than 14 days as compared to the pulsed CO_2 laser, with which 3 to 4 months of erythema are typically noted. The long-term effect on coarse facial rhytides with the Er/YAG laser is undetermined. Although superficially situated epidermal and dermal pathology might respond to the Er/YAG laser, the long-term effect on deep dermal pathology (coarse facial rhytides) is unknown.

Since the Er/YAG laser is associated with a limited depth of penetration, it is well tolerated clinically and does not require sedation or nerve blocks. Most patients can tolerate resurfacing if the skin is pretreated with EMLA 45 minutes prior to resurfacing.

CHOOSING THE RIGHT LASER

Good results can be obtained with any of the lasers currently available. It is difficult to become versatile with all the available lasers, and we suggest that physicians who are planning to buy a laser spend the time to familiarize themselves with the attributes of each machine. We have chosen the Coherent system for our office because of the precision associated with this instrument. Specifically, the collimated handpiece allows consistent fluence delivery to tissue despite the distance the handpiece is held from facial skin. Similarly, the CPG scanner ensures accurate control of spot size overlap and has improved the consistency of results in our practice.

However, we have observed wonderful results after resurfacing with the Sharplan laser. As long as the physician can control the fluence delivered to facial skin (whatever instrument is used) and is experienced in reading the depth of penetration, either of these laser technologies can provide satisfactory results. The decreased expense of the Sharplan system obviously is an important factor, especially for physicians in solo practice.

As important as choosing the proper machine is getting appropriate training in the use of these instruments. Before you purchase a laser, we recommend that you attend one of the numerous laser courses available and then arrange to visit an experienced physician's office and observe laser resurfacing in a number of patients. This allows the novice to determine the settings and number of passes needed to treat specific types of pathology exhibited in photoaged skin. The laser settings for particular areas of the face, the number of passes required to adequately ablate facial rhytides, and reading the depth of penetration (in terms of color changes per pass) cannot be learned from textbooks or teaching courses. Only through a preceptorship with an experienced physician can one learn how to use the laser safely and predictably.

We would urge conservatism when first beginning to perform laser resurfacing. Using lower pulse energy levels and fewer passes is warranted until one becomes skillful in judging the depth of laser penetration. It is far better to perform secondary resurfacing than to place a patient at risk for hypertrophic scarring. As experience is gained, more aggressive resurfacing of deep dermal pathology can be undertaken.

Safety and FDA Compliance*

Lasers are powerful instruments that must be respected. If appropriate safety measures are not adhered to, these machines are capable of inflicting serious injury to physicians, operating room personnel, and the patients they are intended to benefit. The following guidelines should be strictly enforced.

Ocular Protection

1. Never look directly into the CO_2 or helium-neon laser light source or scattered laser light from reflective surfaces. Never look directly into the articulated arm or delivery system laser aperture. Severe eye damage could occur.

2. Because the CO_2 laser beam is highly absorbed by water, the cornea and sclera are the predominant ocular structures at risk for injury and may suffer irreversible damage and scarring as a result of direct or indirect exposure to the CO_2 beam. The severity of injury to these structures depends on how concentrated or diffuse the beam is and the length of exposure time.

3. As a precaution against accidental CO_2 laser exposure to the output beam or its reflection, all persons within the treatment area should wear protective glasses with side shields or goggles as per ANSI recommendations.

4. Laser safety eyewear is not necessary when viewing through a microscope, colposcope, or magnifying loupes because the optics protect the operator's eyes.

5. Glass prescription glasses can be shattered by a high-power density beam.

6. Eye protection for the patient must be provided. Depending on the procedure site, laser safety glasses or one of the following moistened with a nonflammable solution should be used: thick cloths, eye pads, or gauze (4 × 4 inch). If laser surgery is to be performed on the eyelid, metallic, dulled eye shields must be used to protect the eye.

7. The treatment room door should be kept closed during operation of the laser. Glass windows provide sufficient protection from CO_2 laser energy to persons outside the operating room.

8. An ANSI-compliant warning sign should be put on the outside of the treatment room door when the laser is in use to alert personnel before they enter the controlled area. Protective eyewear may be placed outside the treatment room door for personnel to put on before entering the room.

9. Door interlocks may be used to automatically disable the laser when the treatment room door is opened.

*Excerpted from safety guidelines published by Coherent Corporation.

Reflection Hazards

Smooth objects will reflect the laser beam. Reflection hazards can exist several feet beyond the laser beam aperture.

Avoid directing the laser beam at unintended objects. Regardless of the color of a surface, reflection is a potential hazard when the laser strikes a nonabsorbing surface such as a metallic surgical instrument. Use low or nonreflecting instruments whenever possible.

Specular (mirror-like) reflection occurs when the size of surface irregularities is less than the wavelength of the incident light. In this instance the laser beam reflects at the same angles as the angle of incidence. The danger occurs when a concentrated beam of reflected laser light accidently strikes unintended tissue and/or the eyes, causing thermal damage.

Diffuse reflection occurs when surface irregularities are randomly oriented and are much greater than the wavelength of the incident light. In this instance the reflected laser beam is disorganized and scatters in many directions. The laser light may still strike an unintended target surface but the power density will be reduced to a degree that will cause minimal if any thermal effect.

Surgical instruments that will be used in close proximity to the laser beam should be dulled so they are diffusely reflecting. A smooth blackened surface will still specularly reflect the laser beam.

Some equipment manufacturers will dull the surface of your existing surgical instrumentation for use in laser surgery. It is important to consider the composition of your current instrumentation and how the dulling process will affect it (i.e., will it damage the instrument?). Generally, treatment consists of sandblasting the instruments to dull the surface and then possibly ebonizing them with a black finish.

Electrical Hazards

1. Never remove the laser console protective covers. Removing the covers will expose high-voltage components, laser tubes, and possible laser radiation.
2. The area around the laser and footswitch should be kept dry.
3. Never operate the laser if there is any leakage of water from the console.
4. Do not operate the laser if the power cable is faulty or frayed.
5. The laser should undergo routine inspection and maintenance.
6. Extension cords should never be used to operate the laser. A dedicated electrical outlet of appropriate current and amperage is suggested.

Pollution Hazards

1. The laser plume obscures the operative field and is noxious to those who come into direct contact with it. The content of the CO_2 laser plume is currently under investigation. Most investigators agree, from an occupational safety standpoint, that the plume presents a possible pollution hazard. The plume should be effectively evacuated.
2. Repeated suctioning of the laser plume into standard hospital wall suction systems may eventually result in clogging of that system, requiring extensive repair. For minor procedures, wall suction may be used; however, first install an in-line disposable filter.
3. Special in-line vacuum systems designed for evacuation of the laser plume may be installed. Flow capabilities should be adequate to effectively remove the laser plume.
4. A commercial smoke evacuator designed for surgical lasers may be used; these are usually most effective when the plume is extensive. The vacuum tubing or probe used to evacuate the laser plume should not be used to suction blood or fluids unless it is specifically designed and set up to perform both functions simultaneously.

Fire Hazards

1. Never operate the CO_2 surgical laser in the presence of flammable anesthetics, flammable prepping solutions, or other flammable materials. An explosion and/or fire could occur.
2. A CO_2 laser beam can ignite most nonmetallic materials. Use fire-retardant drapes and gowns. The area around the target site can be protected with wet towels or gauze sponges. If allowed to dry, these protective towels and sponges can increase the potential fire hazard. A UL-approved fire extinguisher and water should be readily available.
3. Plastic instrumentation such as speculums or eye shields may melt when impacted by the laser beam, possibly resulting in chemical burns.

Protecting Nontarget Tissues

1. Except during actual treatment, the system must always be in the standby mode. Maintaining the system in the standby mode prevents accidental laser exposure if the footswitch is inadvertently depressed.

2. Always verify that the helium-neon (HeNe) aiming beam and CO_2 laser are aligned before beginning an operative procedure. If the HeNe and CO_2 beams are not aligned, do not use the laser until alignment is corrected.

3. Never make laser treatment exposures if the HeNe aiming beam is not in the field of view. (If the HeNe beam is absent, first make sure that the manual safety shutter is open.)

4. To prevent accidental laser discharge, always turn the system off before installing the delivery system.

5. Never place hands or other objects in the path of the CO_2 beam. Severe burns could occur.

6. Only the person directing the aim of the laser beam should have access to the laser footswitch.

7. Use caution depressing the footswitch when it is in proximity to footswitches for other procedures, such as electrocautery. Make sure the footswitch depressed is the correct one to avoid accidental laser exposure.

8. Never discharge the laser without a target to absorb it and without consideration given to what lies behind the target. It may be desirable to place energy-absorbing material behind a target area when aiming the laser at an oblique target that has healthy tissue as a background. Nontarget tissues may be protected in a variety of ways.
   a. Saline-soaked gauze sponges, moistened cotton-tipped applicators, quartz rods, or titanium rods may be used as backstops for the laser beam. (However, a high-power density laser beam may cause surface splintering of a quartz rod.)
   b. Saline solution may be used in the abdomen to absorb stray laser energy.
   c. Specialized instrumentation such as laparoscopes with laser beam backstops and retractors designed to protect nontarget tissues may be used.
   d. Patients' lips can be protected by moist gauze. When operating in the oral cavity, care should be taken to protect teeth and bones by using wet gauze or other nonflammable, heat-absorbing protective material.

9. Char (carbon debris) may occur with use of the CO_2 laser. However, anhydrous carbon rapidly reaches very high temperatures as laser energy continues to be applied. Heat will then be transferred to adjacent tissues by conduction, resulting in a less controlled thermal effect. When desired, char can be removed by intermittently wiping the treatment surface with gauze sponges or cotton-tipped applicators moistened with water, saline solution, or Ringer's lactate.

10. When anesthesia or pain medication is not used, the comfort and pain tolerance of the patient must be assessed. Unexpected movement by the patient could result in laser exposure to unintended tissue.

Airway Precautions

1. Use of the laser in the presence of oxygen increases the potential fire hazard. When performing a laser procedure in the vicinity of an endotracheal tube, the surgeon and anesthesiologist should carefully select the most appropriate means of airway management.
2. When choosing endotracheal tubes, consider what the by-products of tube combustion are. They should pose the least potential hazard to the patient.
3. Red rubber or silicone endotracheal tubes wrapped with FDA-approved wrapping are commonly used. If using this wrapping, always ensure that the wrapping is removed intact when the patient is extubated.
4. Laser-resistant and cuffed flexible stainless steel endotracheal tubes are commercially available.
5. The endotracheal tube may be further protected by strategic placement of wet sponges to absorb stray laser energy. Ensure that the sponges do not dry and increase the overall fire hazard.
6. The endotracheal tube cuff may be inflated with normal saline solution to protect it from inadvertent penetration. The saline solution may be dyed with methylene blue so evidence of cuff penetration by the laser beam will readily appear on surrounding gauze sponges.
7. Oxygen concentrations should be as low as clinically permissible during airway laser procedures.
8. Anesthetic gases should be least supportive of combustion.

Emergency Laser Shutdown

In the event of an emergency (laser or nonlaser related) the laser should be shut down immediately by depressing the emergency off push button. Some criteria for emergency laser shutdown include:

- Fire
- Faulty shutter operation
- Unauthorized use of the laser
- Misuse of the laser

REFERENCES

Alster TS, Apfelberg DB. Cosmetic Laser Surgery. New York: Wiley-Liss, 1996.

American National Standards Institute. American National Standards for the Safe Use of Lasers in Health Care Facilities. Standard Z136.3-1988. New York: ANSI Publications, 1988.

Apfelberg DB. UltraPulse carbon dioxide laser with CPG scanner for full-face resurfacing for rhytids, photoaging, and acne scars. Plast Reconstr Surg 99:1817, 1997.

Burns AJ. Laser biophysics and laser resurfacing. Course on Cosmetic Laser Applications: Laserbrasion. Presented at the ASPRS Annual Scientific Meeting, Montreal, Oct. 7-11, 1995.

Fitzpatrick RE. Use of the UltraPulse CO_2 laser for dermatology including facial resurfacing. In American Society for Laser Medicine and Surgery Abstracts (Abst. 234). New York: Wiley-Liss, 1995.

Fitzpatrick RE. Depth of varporate and residual thermal damage using multiple passes of the UltraPulse CO_2 laser. In American Society for Laser Medicine and Surgery Abstracts (Abst. 143). New York: Wiley-Liss, 1997.

Fitzpatrick RE, Ruiz-Esparza J, Goldman MP. The depth of thermal necrosis using the CO_2 laser: A comparison of the superpulsed mode and conventional mode. J Dermatol Surg Oncol 17:340, 1991.

Goldman MP, Fitzpatrick RE. Cutaneous Laser Surgery: The Art and Science of Selective Photothermolysis. St. Louis: Mosby–Year Book, 1994.

Hobbs ER, Bailin PL, Wheeland RG, Ratz JL. Superpulsed lasers: Minimizing thermal damage with short duration, high irradiance pulses. J Dermatol Surg Oncol 13:9, 1987.

Lowe NJ, Lask G, Griffin ME, et al. Skin resurfacing with the UltraPulse carbon dioxide laser. J Dermatol Surg 21:1025, 1995.

Ross EV, Grossman MC, Anderson RR, et al. Treatment of facial rhytides: Comparing a pulsed CO_2 laser with a collimated beam to a CO_2 laser enhanced by a flashscanner. In American Society for Laser Medicine and Surgery Abstracts (Abst. 235). New York: Wiley-Liss, 1995.

Seckel BR. Aesthetic Laser Surgery. Boston: Little, Brown, 1996.

Trost D, Zacherl A, Smith MFW. Surgical laser properties and their tissue interaction. In Smith MFW, McEneen JT Jr, eds. Neurological Surgery of the Ear. St. Louis: Mosby, 1992, pp 131-162.

Walsh JT Jr, Deutsch TF. Pulsed CO_2 laser tissue ablation: Measurement of the ablation rate. Lasers Surg Med 8:264, 1988.

Walsh JT Jr, Flotte TJ, Anderson RR, Deutsch TF. Pulsed CO_2 laser tissue ablation: Effect of tissue type and pulse duration on thermal damage. Lasers Surg Med 8:108, 1988.

Weinstein C. Ultrapulsed carbon dioxide laser resurfacing of facial skin for rhytids, scars, and exophytic lessons. Unpublished data, 1997.

Weinstein C, Roberts III TL. Aesthetic skin resurfacing with the high-energy ultrapulsed CO_2 laser. Clin Plast Surg 24:379, 1997.

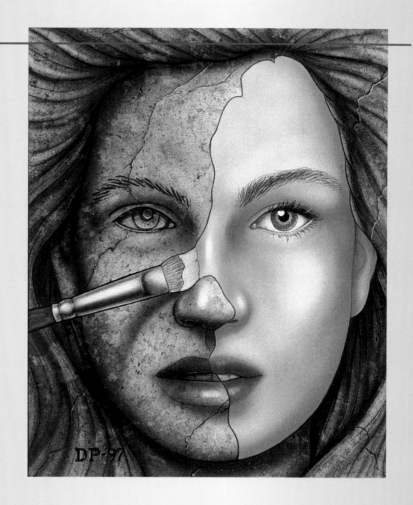

Laser Resurfacing

Laser resurfacing has captured the imagination of physicians, the media, and patients alike. The word "laser" conjures up the image of someone waving a wand to miraculously transform an aged face into a smooth, unblemished, youthful-appearing countenance. Patients who shunned chemical peel are attracted to this "scarless" rejuvenation procedure and are requesting this treatment in record numbers. The remarkable consumer demand for laser rejuvenation is difficult to understand considering that laser resurfacing is associated with a longer recovery time than any facial surgical procedure we perform and the morbidity is similar to that of other deep resurfacing procedures. Since patients often have unrealistic expectations about what lasers can do, they must be informed that laser resurfacing is not a panacea for the aging face, that it is not the "painless" procedure they have been led to believe, and that they must anticipate prolonged posttreatment erythema and the limitations it imposes. However, the advantages are not to be discounted. This modality permits deep peeling in patients who were not candidates for phenol peeling, and the consistency and safety of the results that can now be obtained with the CO_2 laser are so impressive that laser resurfacing is rapidly replacing phenol peeling for the treatment of coarse facial rhytides.

The CO_2 laser is an ideal tool for deep regional resurfacing because of the limited pigmentary and textural changes it produces, making it applicable not only for fair-skinned individuals but for patients with Fitzpatrick types III and IV skin as well. The pulsed CO_2 laser can also be used in conjunction with surgical rejuvenation of the aging face. One of the primary uses of laser therapy is as an adjunct to transconjunctival blepharoplasty for resurfacing the lower eyelid skin, producing results that heretofore were not possible. It can also be used in conjunction with endoscopic forehead plasty to eliminate transverse rhytides and achieve a smooth, unlined forehead. Full-face resurfacing subsequent to face-lift procedures enhances the final result, producing a youthful-appearing skin overlying a surgically corrected foundation. Surgery combined with laser treatment has set a new standard in facial rejuvenation.

HISTOLOGIC CHANGES

The high-energy pulsed CO_2 laser produces a controlled thermal injury that extends through the epidermis and into the papillary and upper reticular dermis. The degree of penetration can be varied according to the depth of the dermatologic pathology and the facial region being treated. Histologic changes following healing show a consistent improvement in epidermal morphology, including epidermal thickening, correction of epidermal atypia, and a return of vertical polarity with cellular maturation.

Changes following laser resurfacing are predicated on the degree of dermal penetration. Once the wound heals, laser injury into the upper reticular dermis stimulates fibroplasia and angiogenesis that results in neocollagen formation and regeneration of dermal elastic fibers. Biopsies show that epidermal healing is complete 2 weeks following laser resurfacing, although dermal changes persist for as long as 6 months. Biopsies performed 2 weeks following laser injury demonstrate marked fibroplasia, and biopsies demonstrate significant neocollagen formation 3 months following resurfacing as well as a diminution in dermal glycosaminoglycans, which are typically found in degenerated elastotic dermis. Biopsies performed 6 months following resurfacing show stable collagen formation.

The histologic changes following laser resurfacing parallel those of phenol peeling. The major difference between these two treatment modalities is seen at the level of epidermal melanocytes. Epidermal melanocytes are present after phenol peeling but no longer have the ability to synthesize melanin; epidermal melanocytes are evenly dispersed along the basement membrane of the epidermis after laser resurfacing and retain their ability to function. This finding has even been confirmed in biopsies performed on black skin, showing a return of normal melanocytic function 3 months after laser resurfacing.

Although laser resurfacing appears to be less detrimental to melanocyte function than phenol peeling, as with all resurfacing modalities, the deeper the laser penetrates, the higher the risk of hypopigmentation. However, if hypopigmentation does occur subsequent to laser treatment, it tends to be less severe than with other techniques. Clinically, deeper laser resurfacing for coarse facial rhytides is associated with a greater risk of pigmentary changes (see Chapter 2 for more details).

INDICATIONS

Similar to other deep resurfacing agents, laser resurfacing is indicated in patients presenting with dermatologic problems localized to the reticular dermis. We have used lasers primarily to treat facial wrinkling and to improve the appearance of acne scarring. It is also an effective method for treating severe facial dyschromias.

Photoaged Skin and Rhytides

Both coarse and fine facial wrinkling are amenable to laser treatment. Not only does surface texture improve, but the face appears intrinsically tighter secondary to regeneration of dermal collagen and elastic fibers. Patients appear rejuvenated because their facial skin has the histologic and morphologic attributes of young skin.

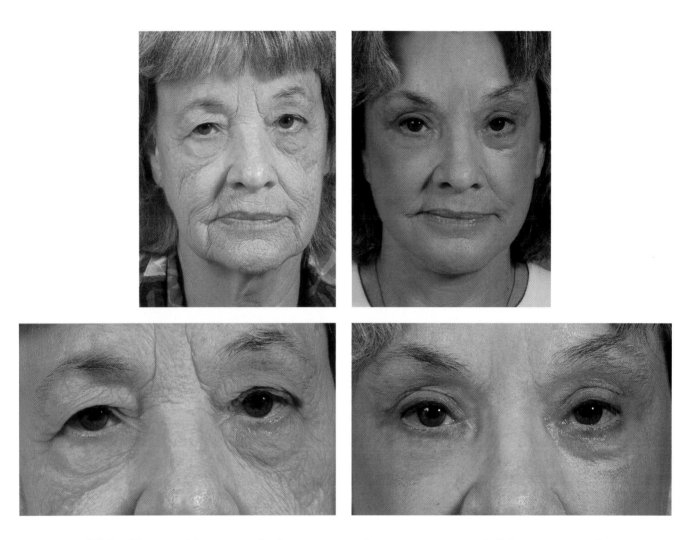

This 67–year–old woman had severe sun damage accompanied by coarse and fine facial rhytides. She is shown following an upper and lower blepharoplasty, forehead plasty, rhytidectomy, and subsequent full–face laser resurfacing. Treatment of the gravitational changes of aging in conjunction with correction of the intrinsic damage associated with photoaged skin produces a result not attainable with a single treatment modality.

Epidermal Dysplasias

Patients with severe actinic damage in association with epidermal dysplasia and multiple actinic keratoses can also benefit from laser resurfacing. The ablation of the dysplastic epidermis following laser treatment and the resulting normal–appearing epidermis that regenerates on healing significantly improve the quality of the damaged skin in these patients. The results are comparable to those obtained with phenol peeling.

Acne Scarring

Dermabrasion has been the traditional approach for treating acne scars. In the past 2 years we have used laser resurfacing to treat these difficult problems. As with dermabrasion, the results following laser resurfacing of acne scars are less than perfect, but the patient usually can expect improvement, and in our opinion patient satisfaction is somewhat higher than with dermabrasion.

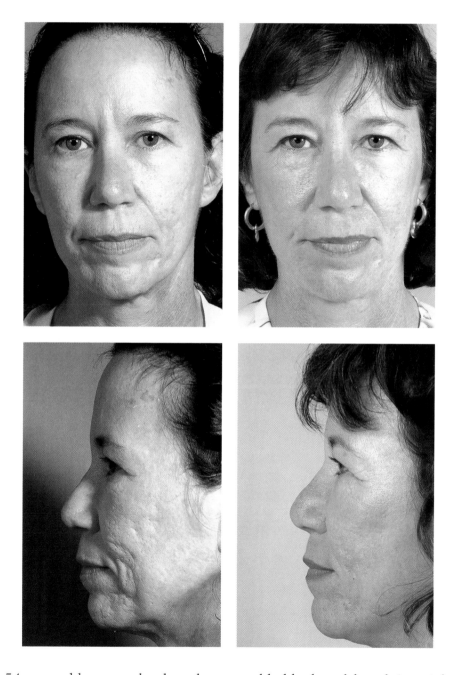

This 54-year-old woman has long been troubled by broad-based, ice-pick-type acne scars. She is shown 14 months after full-face laser resurfacing. Although the acne scars are still visible, they are less noticeable. Note the general improvement in skin tone. Her facial skin appears tighter and enhances the overall result.

Dyschromia

Most disorders of facial pigmentation can be treated using superficial or medium-depth peeling in conjunction with a skin care regimen. Only rarely is deep resurfacing necessary to treat pigmentary problems. One of the added benefits of laser resurfacing is that clumping of pigment along the basement membrane of the epidermis resolves with epidermal regeneration, ameliorating the typical dyschromia associated with photoaging. Patients who have facial pigmentation disorders and other problems associated with prolonged sun exposure will show an improvement.

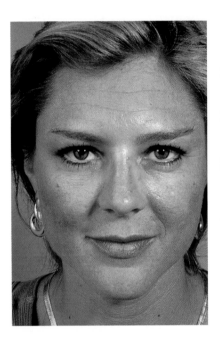 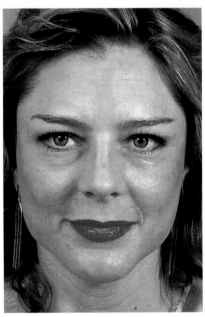

This 30-year-old woman requested laser resurfacing to improve her sun-damaged skin and treat mild acne scarring. She is shown 6 months following full-face resurfacing. Although the acne scars are not significantly improved, the severe dyschromia resulting from previous actinic exposure is eliminated. Deep resurfacing in conjunction with daily sunscreens, sun avoidance, and strict adherence to a skin care regimen will commonly eliminate the pigmentation resulting from photoaging.

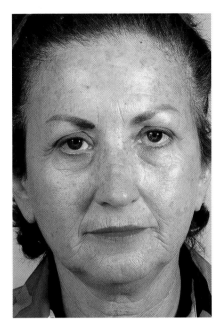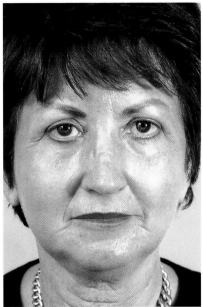

Prolonged actinic exposure resulted in facial rhytides and a mottled complexion in this middle-aged woman. Full-face resurfacing ameliorated the wrinkles, uniformly lightened the facial pigmentation, and eliminated the blotchiness. Use of Retin-A and hydroquinone and sun avoidance have helped maintain the result.

PATIENT SELECTION

Unlike phenol peels or dermabrasion, laser resurfacing is applicable to a wide variety of patients. Although our experience with laser resurfacing has largely been in patients with Fitzpatrick types I to III skin because these patients are most susceptible to photoaging, we have successfully treated patients with type IV skin. Postinflammatory pigmentation is a possibility in all patients undergoing deep resurfacing, although patients with dark complexions are at greater risk. Pre- and posttreatment skin care regimens to suppress melanin production are essential to ensure healing with uniform pigmentation. Sun avoidance, sunscreens, and covering cosmetics are also critical during the recovery period.

At the present time we have not performed laser resurfacing in patients with Fitzpatrick types V and VI facial skin. Although our histologic studies on black skin suggest that resurfacing can be done safely, clinical studies have not yet been performed. Both postinflammatory hyperpigmentation and hypopigmentation are of concern in this patient population.

Hyperpigmentation subsequent to resurfacing is troublesome; however, unlike hypopigmentation, it can be treated. Our experience suggests that hypopigmentation is most likely to develop in patients with Fitzpatrick types I and II skin and is more noticeable following regional resurfacing. Fair-skinned individuals are prone to hypopigmentation because there is less pigment in the epidermis to camouflage the dermal changes that occur with resurfacing. The epidermis is translucent, making the underlying dermal changes more obvious. The incidence of pigmentary changes after laser treatment is lower than that observed after phenol peeling or dermabrasion, and when it does occur, it tends to be milder. Patients with coarse rhytides appear to be at greatest risk since deeper laser penetration is necessary. The deeper the resurfacing into the dermis, the more likely hypopigmentation will result. If hypopigmentation is of concern to a patient, it may be wise to limit the depth of resurfacing during the initial application. Residual rhytides can be treated as a secondary touch-up at a later date.

INSTRUCTIONS TO PATIENTS

An informed patient with realistic expectations is essential to ensure a smooth postoperative course. Many patients mistakenly believe that laser resurfacing is a "quick fix." The recovery period following full-face laser resurfacing is similar to that for phenol peeling—7 to 10 days for open wounds to reepithelialize and 8 to 12 weeks of posttreatment erythema that requires the use of covering cosmetics to conceal. The recovery period after full-face laser resurfacing is longer than for most facial aesthetic surgical procedures. The morbidity and postoperative recovery should be thoroughly discussed to promote patient compliance and uneventful healing. Written instruction sheets are helpful.

TECHNIQUE
Prelaser Skin Care Regimen

We treat all patients undergoing laser resurfacing with 0.1% Retin-A and 4% hydroquinone prior to the procedure. In patients with types I and II skin the regimen is begun 2 weeks preoperatively and in those with darker complexions 4 to 8 weeks prior to resurfacing. Pretreatment with Retin-A and hydroquinone offers several advantages. Inhibiting melanin synthesis prior to resurfacing provides greater control of postpeel pigmentation. We have observed that patients pretreated with Retin-A undergo reepithelialization more quickly than those who have not. Pretreatment conditions patients to use the creams properly and reinforces postoperative compliance. Most patients will develop blotchy pigmentation after laser resurfacing if a proper skin care routine is not followed.

Antiviral and Antibacterial Prophylaxis

As with other deep resurfacing procedures, herpes simplex infection can occur after laser resurfacing in patients who harbor this virus. Approximately 6% to 10% of patients with a negative herpes simplex virus history will develop an infection after reticular dermal resurfacing. For this reason, we treat all of our

Patient Instructions for Laser Resurfacing

Before Treatment

- Your face will be thoroughly cleansed to remove all residue and makeup.

- You will be given a mild sedative by mouth approximately 15 minutes before the procedure to induce relaxation. Prior to the procedure you will be given an intravenous anesthetic by our board-certified anesthesiologist. You will experience no pain or discomfort during the procedure.

After Treatment

- Your face will be swollen and there will be some oozing in the areas treated for 24 to 48 hours following laser resurfacing. Discomfort is common during this period and you will be given pain medication that can be taken as necessary. For mild pain, extra-strength Tylenol is recommended.

- You will be expected to cleanse your face four times a day with a washcloth or gauze sponges and cool tap water on the first day after treatment. You must carefully remove any secretions as well as ointment and then reapply a greasy cleansing ointment. You can take a shower but soap should not be allowed to contact the laser-treated areas. This process is repeated until wound healing is completed, usually within 7 to 10 days.

- The treated areas will go through a crusting phase, which can make cleansing difficult. If you are unable to adequately care for your wounds, please request assistance.

- When the crusting has resolved, the fresh new skin will have a pink color, but this will fade over a period of 8 to 12 weeks. During this time covering cosmetics, sunscreens, and sun avoidance are essential.

- Two weeks following laser resurfacing you must resume every-other-night application of Retin-A and hydroquinone to laser-treated areas. Since your skin will be sensitive at first, apply these creams lightly until the skin adjusts, at which time the applications are made nightly until all redness has faded. If your skin is sensitive to Retin-A, a pigmentation cream containing kojic acid and hydroquinone may be substituted.

patients undergoing laser resurfacing with either prophylactic acyclovir (400 mg three times a day for 5 days) or with valacyclovir (500 mg twice a day) beginning 24 hours preoperatively. Since adopting this policy we have seen no case of herpes infection.

Although bacterial infection is unusual after partial-thickness skin resurfacing, the potential remains for postoperative infection to convert a partial-thickness injury to a full-thickness one. We routinely use a 5-day course of antibiotics (keflex, 250 mg four times a day) to prevent this potential problem. Frequent inspection of the resurfaced skin as well as meticulous postoperative wound care will help minimize this problem.

Patient Preparation and Safety Considerations

The patient is marked for laser resurfacing while upright. If regional resurfacing is to be performed, such as in the lower eyelid or perioral areas, these are marked. Deep lines requiring special attention are outlined. If full-face resurfacing is to be performed, the mandibular border is marked so that cervical skin is left undisturbed and the resulting line of demarcation camouflaged. Resurfacing of the neck is unpredictable and risky. Since cervical skin has only 10% of the adnexal structures found in facial skin, healing following deep resurfacing can be slow.

We use intravenous sedatives for most of our patients undergoing laser resurfacing in conjunction with nerve blocks and local infiltration of facial skin. If a small area of skin is to be resurfaced regionally, local blocks are adequate without the use of sedation. Topically applied EMLA cream helps diminish the pain associated with local anesthetic infiltration. For anesthetic induction, we typically use midazolam and ketamine, but a propofol drip can be used as well. If patients experience pain during resurfacing after regional and local field blockade, narcotics (fentanyl) and minor tranquilizers (midazolam) can be used to supplement the sedation. Any patient undergoing intravenous sedation must be properly monitored.

After the local anesthetic has been infiltrated, we apply tetracaine eyedrops so that the laser eye shield can be inserted. Protection of the globe is of utmost importance before resurfacing the periorbital region.

The facial skin is washed with normal saline solution and a mild soap and then thoroughly dried. The skin must be dry since the CO_2 laser will not penetrate water. To prevent intraoperative fires, the patient's hair and the surrounding regions not to be treated are draped in wet towels or aluminum foil. The patient's teeth are protected with a moist gauze sponge to prevent injury of the dental enamel when resurfacing the perioral region. No supplemental oxygen is used to reduce fire hazards. Before the laser is turned on, operating room personnel are instructed to don the proper eye gear and the smoke evacuator is activated to remove the laser plume.

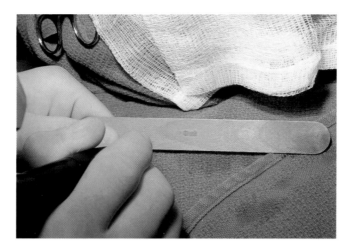

The 3 mm Truespot handpiece is tested on a moist tongue blade prior to laser delivery to facial skin.

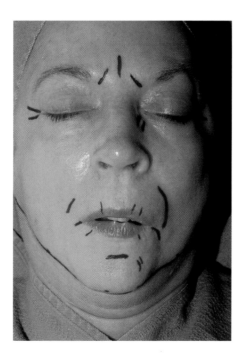

Preoperative markings are made with the patient in the sitting position prior to sedation. Coarse rhytides are inked and the mandibular border delineated.

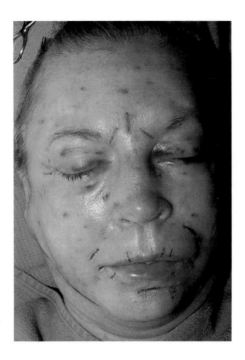

Following administration of the intravenous anesthetic and infiltration of a local anesthetic solution the deep rhytides are resurfaced with a single pass of the 3 mm handpiece at 500 mJ. This initial pass is preliminary to later resurfacing with the computerized pattern generator (CPG) scanner to facilitate more complete correction.

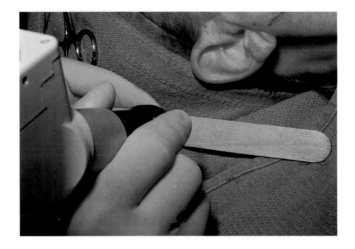

The CPG scanner is tested on a moist tongue blade prior to laser delivery to facial skin.

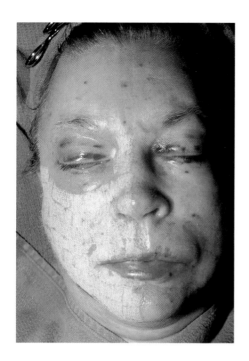

The patient is seen following a single pass of the CPG scanner (300 mJ with a density of 6) to the cheek skin on the right. The right forehead and periorbital area have been resurfaced (density of 6 × 2 passes for the forehead; density of 5 × 2 passes for the upper and lower eyelids). Note that the ocular protector is in place.

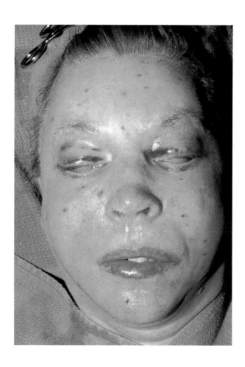

At the end of the procedure the patient's skin appears smooth, tightened, and uniform in color and texture. The eyebrows seem to be positioned higher since the forehead skin is tightened by the laser treatment. In addition, the cheek skin looks firmer and the jowls reduced. This is the clinical end point that we wish to obtain. Although resurfacing could have been carried deeper (to the point where the skin turns to a brown or chamois color), it is unnecessary; an extra pass with the laser will have little benefit and will increase the chance of posttreatment hypopigmentation.

Intraoperative Decision Making

When planning laser resurfacing, the pulse energy and number of passes must be determined. In general increasing the pulse energy and increasing the number of passes will result in a greater degree of dermal penetration.

A higher pulse energy results in more complete vaporization and ablation of tissue; a lower pulse energy results in less tissue vaporization but is more commonly associated with conductive thermal injury. For this reason, we typically set the machine at high levels of pulse energy to ensure adequate vaporization secondary to optical penetration while attempting to minimize conductive heat delivery. This allows greater precision in resurfacing and lessens the number of passes.

We favor the Coherent UltraPulse laser because the laser beam is collimated so that the distance of the handpiece from facial skin does not affect the amount of energy delivered. The availability of the CPG scanner allows the use of a multitude of sizes and shapes of preset patterns that correspond to the areas being treated, making laser resurfacing more rapid. In our opinion the precision and safety of laser resurfacing are enhanced by the use of the CPG scanner because it minimizes human error. This scanning device allows the physician to control the spot size overlap or "density" of the laser energy delivered; density can be varied from 0.0% to 60% (density settings of 1 to 9). Rather than varying pulse energy (which we usually keep at a maximum level of 300 mJ) we adjust laser penetration by varying the density of spot overlap. In other words, in an area that does not require deep resurfacing a density of 3 to 4 will result in less penetration, whereas a density of 6 to 7 will result in more profound resurfacing (similar to phenol penetration depending on the number of passes). We typically use a density overlap of 30% to 35% (density of 5 to 6) in resurfacing patients with coarse facial rhytides.

The number of passes applied to facial skin is key to obtaining consistent results. Thin skin will not tolerate as many passes as thick, oily skin. Patients with acne scarring often need more passes than elderly patients with thin, dry skin. Similarly, resurfacing of the lower eyelid will require fewer passes than resurfacing of deeply wrinkled, thick forehead skin.

Laser Delivery

We approach laser delivery in a regional fashion. The deepest rhytides are resurfaced with a single pass of the 3 mm Truespot handpiece at the beginning of the procedure. We then resurface the periorbital region using either the 3 mm Truespot handpiece or the CPG scanner. The skin directly overlying the pretarsal and preseptal orbicularis is resurfaced at a lower density than the skin overlying the periorbital area as well as crow's-feet (the CPG setting we commonly use for eyelid skin is 300 mJ and a density of 5; we increase the density to 6 for the crow's-feet regions). It is rare that more than two passes are needed to resurface the upper and lower eyelid. In resurfacing the upper eyelid we take care not to apply the laser to the pretarsal skin of the upper lid. Similar to phenol peeling, resurfacing of upper lid pretarsal skin adds little to the result but significantly increases postoperative edema that interferes with eyelid opening. When resurfacing the upper lid, care must be taken not to burn the eyebrow. Similar concern is warranted in resurfacing the inner canthal region to prevent epicanthal webbing postoperatively.

We then proceed to resurface the forehead, glabella, and nasal dorsum. The skin in this region of the face is thick, well endowed with adnexal structures, and less likely to scar. The forehead is resurfaced using the CPG scanner set at 300 mJ and a density typically of 5 or 6. The first pass removes the epidermis and penetrates the upper papillary dermis. The second pass is critical to obtaining the desired result since the laser begins to penetrate the reticular dermis with this pass. Usually two passes of the CPG scanner at the settings noted will effectively resurface the forehead in most patients. In some patients with deep rhytides and thick skin a third pass of the entire region may be warranted depending on the appearance of the skin after the second application.

The cheeks are then resurfaced in much the same fashion as the forehead. Cheek skin is usually responsive to two passes with the laser. Blending the previously treated periorbital and forehead skin is important to produce a uniform result.

We treat the perioral area last during full-face resurfacing. In our experience deep perioral rhytides show an inconsistent response. Most patients can be treated with two passes with the CPG scanner set at a spot density of 6, although initially we pretreat the shoulders of the deep rhytides with the 3 mm handpiece set at 500 mJ. The clinical appearance of perioral skin and the elimination of wrinkling should serve as a guide as to whether a third pass is required.

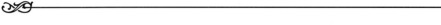

Key Technical Points

- *Magnification:* Since eyewear is required for performing laser resurfacing, we find it helpful to use loupe magnification. Magnification adds precision to resurfacing, allowing visualization of any small remaining rhytides, accurate assessment of spot overlap, and proper reading of skin color following resurfacing. Although not mandatory, magnification is a useful adjunct for obtaining consistent results.

- *Limiting thermal conductive injury:* Although some degree of spot overlap is required in laser resurfacing, too much overlap can lead to the buildup of debris or "char." Char acts as a heat sink, producing high temperatures where the char builds up and resulting in conductive thermal injury to adjacent skin. Experience suggests that depth of penetration should be secondary to optical penetration rather than by conductive thermal injury. Applying repetitive laser pulses to the same region prior to removing char is a technical error, makes reading the depth of penetration of the laser impossible, and can result in postoperative scarring.

- *Removal of debris between passes:* It is essential to remove the debris that results from tissue coagulation following each pass of the laser. For this reason, we prefer to perform full-face resurfacing regionally so that debris can be removed while it is still nonadherent. If the debris is not properly removed, char buildup will occur and cause conductive thermal injury. Moist gauze sponges are useful for removing the necrotic tissue.

- *Dry operative field:* After the laser debris is removed, the operative field must be dried thoroughly before making another pass because the CO_2 laser will not penetrate water.

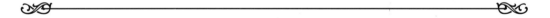

Reading The Laser

Laser resurfacing is a visual art. Understanding the depth of penetration with each pass and the end point of resurfacing is essential. The obvious visual end point is elimination of facial rhytides and the creation of smooth-textured skin. Skin color is the critical landmark in judging depth of penetration. The typical color-change scenario when the CPG scanner is set at 300 mJ and a density of 6 is as follows: The first pass removes the epidermis and penetrates to the level of the papillary dermis and the skin appears pink. The next pass of the laser penetrates into the upper reticular dermis and the skin turns a whitish brown color. The third pass of the laser penetrates deeper into the reticular dermis and typically a chamois-like tan color can be observed. This represents the absolute end point of safe resurfacing. Even if residual rhytides remain, no further resurfacing should be performed once this tan color is observed. It is far safer to subject the patient to a secondary revision than to risk hypertrophic scarring.

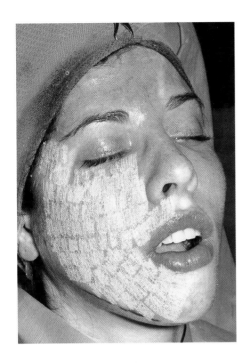

This 25-year-old woman had laser resurfacing for acne scarring on her cheeks. It was necessary to determine how deep to resurface the facial skin that had not been affected by the acne. We elected to treat the unblemished skin with only a single pass to ensure a good color blend. She is shown after a single pass to the forehead (note pink color) before a first pass was made to the right cheek and lower eyelid with a CPG setting of 300 mJ and a density of 6.

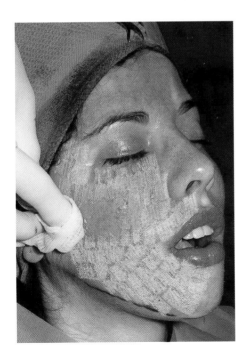

The debris is removed after the first pass with a moist gauze pad. Note the pink color beneath the debris that represents the appearance of the papillar dermis after vaporization of the epidermis.

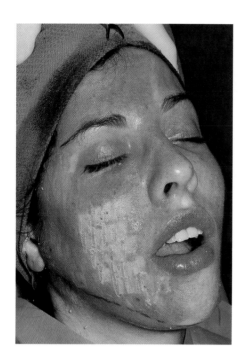

A second pass at the same energy settings is made over areas exhibiting deeper acne scars. A second pass to unblemished facial skin would add little to the final result and increase the risk of hypopigmentation. Postoperative morbidity is decreased by limiting the number of passes.

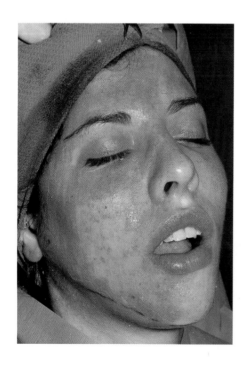

The whitish brown color of the resurfaced skin can be observed when the debris is cleared after the second pass. Note the contrast between the brown color of the upper reticular dermis and the pinker color of the papillary dermis in those areas treated with a single pass. Her facial skin appears smooth. If residual scars are still present, it is safe to perform a third pass since the skin has not assumed the dark brown or chamois color signaling the end point.

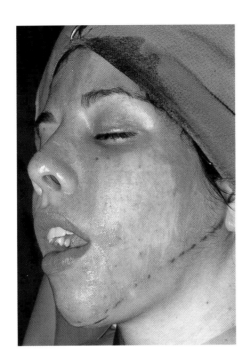

Observe the appearance of the left cheek after two passes over the areas of acne scarring. The color differential after a single pass and two passes is again clearly seen.

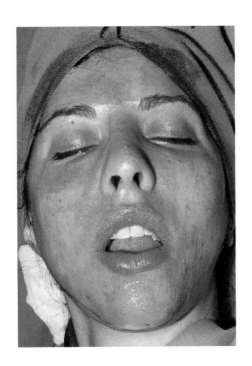

At the end of the procedure the skin appears smooth, and the blending of texture between the areas treated with a single pass and the areas of acne scarring treated with two passes can be seen. There was no need to resurface upper lid skin in this young patient.

IMMEDIATE WOUND CARE

Closed wound dressings (Flexan or Second Skin) are commonly used following full-face laser resurfacing. They are associated with less pain, lack of exudate, and limited crust formation. Many believe these dressings promote earlier re-epithelialization and less erythema. The disadvantages of closed wound dressings are that they are cumbersome to apply, require frequent changing, and are difficult to reapply following removal.

In contrast, open wound care is simple to perform and permits early cleansing of the wound. It also facilitates examination of wounds. Open wound care with frequent application of a Vaseline-based ointment requires greater patient involvement because the wounds must be washed four to five times a day and the ointment reapplied.

The use of occlusive dressings or open wound care is a matter of individual preference and does not affect the result if patients are closely followed. Currently we favor open care using Aquaphor ointment. This emollient is more soothing to the patient than either Vaseline or A & D ointment and is associated with rapid reepithelialization. Our nursing staff monitors patients frequently to ensure that wound care is properly maintained. Reepithelialization typically occurs between 7 and 10 days after treatment, at which point less greasy ointments can be substituted.

If occlusive dressings are to be used, they need to be changed frequently. We have seen two patients with bacterial superinfection and one patient with a *Candida* infection who were referred from other offices where the occlusive dressing was left in place for several days. One of these cases resulted in severe hypertrophic scarring. *Deep resurfacing mandates meticulous wound care to ensure rapid healing.*

LATE POSTOPERATIVE CARE

Greasy ointments are discontinued and lighter ointments substituted after re-epithelialization. Since the sebaceous glands do not function properly for 3 to 5 weeks, some type of moisturizer is usually required. As oil function normalizes, the need for moisturizers can be individualized.

Covering makeup serves two functions: it allows the patient to return to daily activities and provides protection from the sun. Covering cosmetics can be used between 10 days and 2 weeks after the procedure. An office-based aesthetician can help patients select the proper shade of camouflaging makeup to best conceal the erythema.

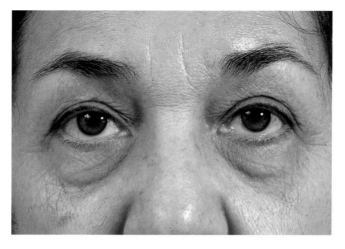

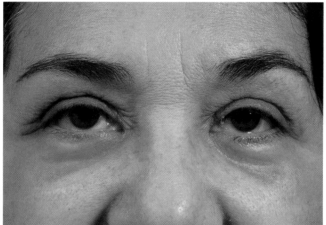

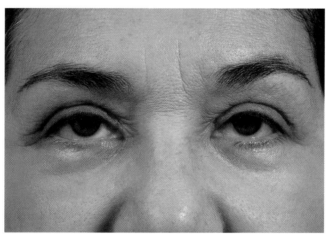

Laser settings: 3 mm Truespot handpiece at 500 mJ × 2 passes

This patient had an upper blepharoplasty, transconjunctival lower blepharoplasty, and laser resurfacing of the lower lids and crow's-feet. Two weeks after treatment reepithelialization has occurred and camouflaging makeup easily covers the erythema, permitting the patient to resume normal activities. The photographs in the middle and below were taken on the same day following application of makeup.

The application of sunscreens to block UVA sunlight is important in preventing posttreatment hyperpigmentation. Sun avoidance is stressed, including wearing hats and sunglasses. As long as erythema is present, such activities as golf, tennis, swimming, and jogging during daylight should be curtailed.

The most important element of postoperative care in preventing postinflammatory hyperpigmentation is reinstitution of the skin care regimen consisting of Retin-A and hydroquinone. These creams are begun on the fourteenth day after resurfacing and are used on an every-other-night basis until the patient can tolerate nightly applications. Since the skin is usually sensitive at this time, it can be difficult to get some patients to adhere to a proper skin care program. Retin-A application will also make posttreatment erythema more obvious, and some patients will stop applying this cream. The importance of preventing postinflammatory hyperpigmentation using a proper skin care regimen cannot be overstressed, and patient compliance is essential to ensure uniform healing. In patients with darker skin types a morning application of kojic acid will help control hyperpigmentation after the nightly application of Retin-A and hydroquinone is tolerated.

RESULTS

Full-face laser resurfacing produces a predictable improvement in the stigmata of photoaging. Both coarse and fine facial rhytides are ameliorated and uniform facial pigmentation obtained. Dynamic facial rhytides associated with animation, such as in the nasolabial fold, glabellar region, and crow's-feet areas, will persist despite aggressive therapy; however, wrinkle lines seen in repose will be improved. It is more difficult to eliminate rhytides along the upper and lower lips. Initially our results in this region were inconsistent as compared with dermabrasion or phenol. As we have gained more experience, especially following the introduction of the CPG scanner, our results have improved.

Unlike phenol peeling, which produces clinical and histologic results that last for up to 20 years, the longevity of results achieved with laser resurfacing has yet to be determined. We have seen several patients in whom the initial results were good, but their rhytides recurred several months later. As we have become more experienced at reading the laser and have performed deeper and more aggressive laser resurfacing when required, the results have become more consistent and longevity has improved.

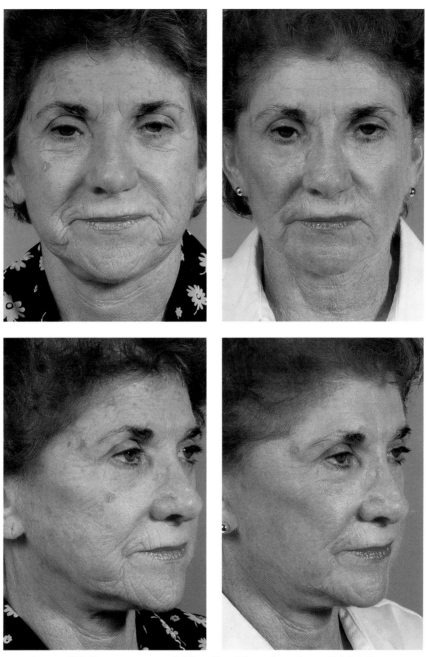

Scanner settings: CPG scanner at 300 mJ with a density of 6 × 2 passes; density of 5 for lower and upper eyelids

This 72-year-old woman had signs of long-standing photodamage. Some years ago she had a face lift and an upper lip phenol peel. Note her fine and coarse facial rhytides and mottled complexion. Seven months after laser resurfacing most of her facial rhytides are eliminated and her skin appears tighter and more youthful. The line of demarcation between treated and untreated skin is obvious on the oblique view. This represents a return to her natural skin color, which is distinctive from the photoaged mottling in the untreated cervical skin. Compare the laser-resurfaced skin with the hypopigmentation of the upper lip resulting from the previous phenol peel. Hypopigmentation from phenol tends to be more severe than that associated with laser resurfacing.

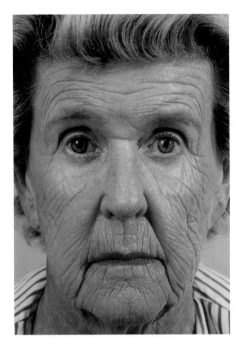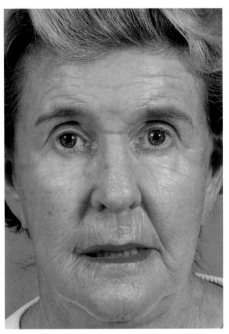

Laser settings: 3 mm Truespot handpiece; 500 mJ × 2 passes for forehead, lower eyelids, and perioral areas; two additional passes at 350 mJ for residual rhytides of forehead and mouth.

Severe actinic exposure in patients with type II skin invariably leads to a weathered appearance and coarse rhytides, as seen in this elderly woman. She underwent rhytidectomy and simultaneous laser resurfacing of the forehead, perioral, and periorbital areas. She is shown 4 months following treatment. The residual perioral erythema reflects the increased depth of penetration required to improve such profound wrinkling.

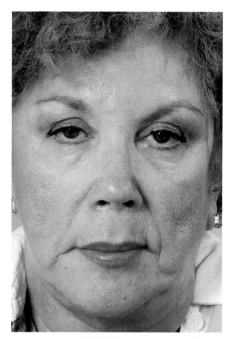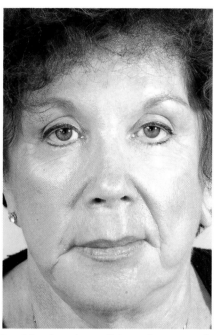

Scanner settings: CPG scanner at 300 mJ with density of 6 × 2 passes for face and forehead; density of 5 × 2 passes for lower and upper eyelids; two additional passes at density of 5 for spot cheek rhytides

This 68-year-old woman has thick, oily skin with a mosaic pattern of facial rhytides. Laser resurfacing was performed with up to four passes to treat her deep cheek wrinkles. Because of the thickness and oiliness of her skin, rapid healing was evident despite the deep level of resurfacing. Five months following treatment skin appearance, texture, and tightening are noticeably improved. No surgical procedure was necessary.

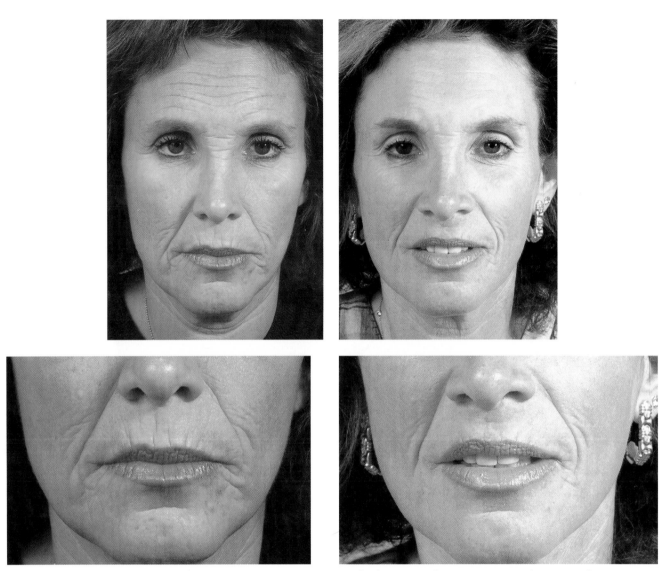

Scanner settings: CPG scanner at 300 mJ with density of 6 × 2 passes; density of 5 × 2 passes for lower and upper eyelids; density of 5 × 2 additional passes for spot areas such as glabella, forehead, and perioral regions

This 50-year-old woman initially requested a face lift. In our judgment photoaging was the primary culprit. She is shown 9 months after full-face laser resurfacing. Prolonged postoperative treatment with Retin-A, hydroquinone, and sun avoidance has helped to maintain the result and improve her blotchy pigmentation.

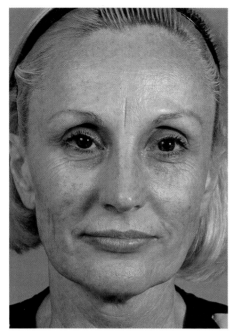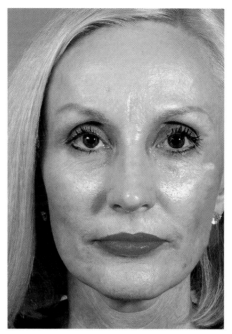

Laser settings: CPG scanner at 300 mJ with density of 6 × 2 passes to face and forehead; density of 5 × 2 passes to upper and lower eyelids

Actinically damaged Fitzpatrick type II facial skin typically appears mottled with coarse and fine rhytides most apparent in the periorbital region. This patient is shown 7 months after full-face resurfacing, which improved her facial rhytides and dyschromia. She exhibits moderate hypopigmentation, which is more commonly seen in patients with this skin type.

REGIONAL LASER RESURFACING COMBINED WITH SURGICAL REJUVENATION

Many physicians believe that segmental treatment produces an inferior clinical result compared with full-face laser resurfacing. Color differences in treated and untreated skin are more apparent following regional treatment. It is also easier for patients to apply camouflaging makeup to the entire face than to conceal isolated facial regions.

Although we agree with these points, the limited pigmentary changes subsequent to laser treatment make it an ideal tool for regional resurfacing. If deep dermal pathology is limited to a specific region of the face, we also believe that resurfacing in areas where sun damage is minimal represents overtreatment. Many patients exhibit both the gravitational affects of aging as well as the stigmata of photoaging. The combination of laser resurfacing with surgical rejuvenation has proved to be consistently effective in these cases.

Laser resurfacing will tighten facial skin; however, it is not a substitute for rhytidectomy. In patients with gravitational changes and coarse rhytides a face lift can be performed and full-face resurfacing delayed until the patient has recovered from surgery. Although undermined facial skin can be resurfaced, conservatism is warranted to minimize the risk of scarring.

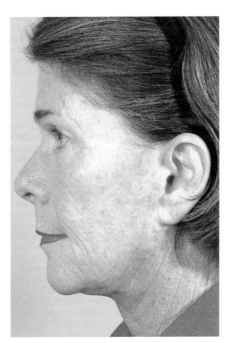 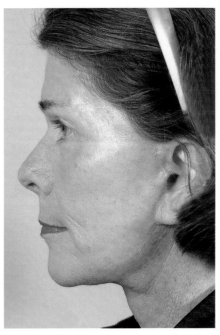

Scanner settings: CPG scanner at 300 mJ; density of 5 × 2 passes for forehead; density of 6 × 1 pass for lower eyelids; density of 6 × 2 passes for perioral region; density of 5 × 1 pass for cheeks

Although we rarely resurface surgically undermined skin, we elected to do so in this patient. When the face lift was completed, we resurfaced the thick facial flaps where surgical undermining was limited using a single pass of the CPG scanner. Caution is advisable in these circumstances, and if there is any doubt, resurfacing should be delayed until healing is complete.

Certain clinical situations lend themselves to a combination of surgery and resurfacing. Laser resurfacing of the forehead in conjunction with an endoscopic brow lift is a safe and efficacious procedure. Similarly, transconjunctival blepharoplasty with laser treatment of the lower eyelids removes herniated lower lid fat and tightens wrinkled lower lid skin. Although we do not hesitate to use laser resurfacing on patients undergoing transconjunctival blepharoplasty, we *never* combine laser resurfacing with transcutaneous blepharoplasty.

Lid tone must be evaluated carefully before deciding to resurface the lower eyelid. If the patient exhibits lower lid laxity or obvious lid retraction, some form of canthoplasty should be performed prior to or at the time of lid resurfacing.

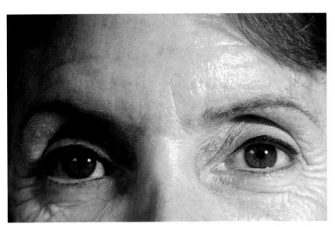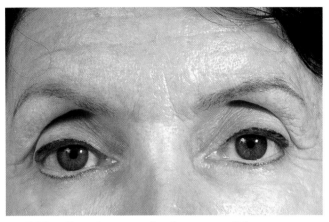

Laser settings: 3 mm Truespot handpiece at 500 mJ × 2 passes for lower eyelids

Deep crow's-feet and lower lid rhytides are a common stigmata of middle age. This patient is shown 1 year following resurfacing of the lower lids and crow's-feet. The slight erythema that can be observed probably is the result of continued daily use of Retin-A and glycolic acid for maintenance therapy.

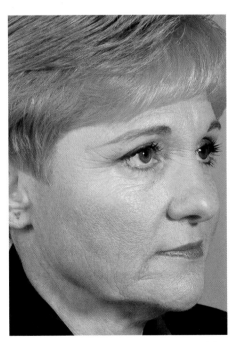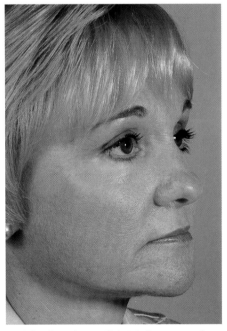

Scanner settings: CPG scanner at 300 mJ with density of 6 × 2 passes for perioral rhytides; 3 mm Truespot handpiece at 500 mJ × 2 passes for lower eyelids

This 55-year-old Hispanic woman has the typical stigmata of actinic exposure and gravitational aging. She is shown 8 months after a face lift, upper blepharoplasty, and laser resurfacing of the periorbital area and mouth. Although there is no obvious line of demarcation following periorbital resurfacing, moderate hypopigmentation is evident in the perioral region.

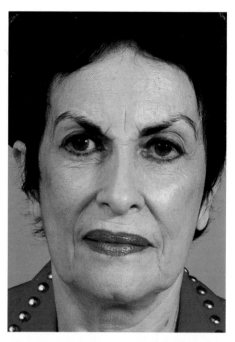

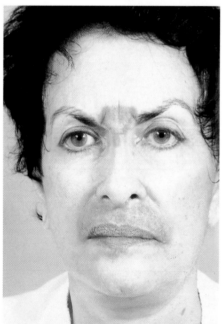
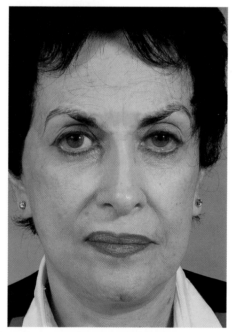

Laser settings: 3 mm Truespot handpiece at 500 mJ × 2 passes

This Hispanic patient with Fitzpatrick type III skin is at risk for postinflammatory pigmentation. She underwent a face lift and laser resurfacing of the glabella and upper lip. She was not placed on a posttreatment skin care regimen. One month after treatment she has significant hyperpigmentation in the laser-treated areas, which was managed by aggressive application of Retin-A, hydroquinone, and kojic acid. Eight months later most of the postinflammatory pigmentation has resolved, although her upper lip now appears hypopigmented compared with the surrounding skin. This patient also exemplifies how difficult it is to camouflage the line of demarcation between treated and untreated skin after any deep resurfacing procedure.

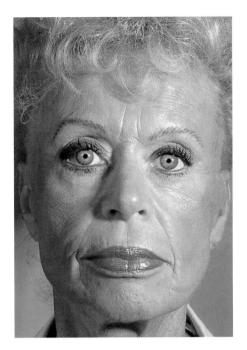

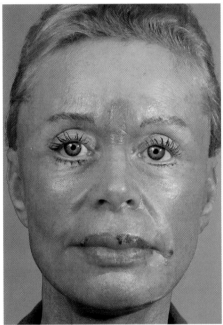
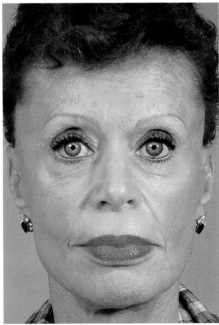

Laser settings: 3 mm Truespot handpiece; 500 mJ × 2 passes for glabella; 400 mJ × 2 passes for lower eyelids; 500 mJ × 2 passes for perioral region

A combination of facial laxity and sun damage is evident in this 56-year-old patient. She had a face lift in conjunction with regional laser resurfacing of the lower eyelids, crow's-feet areas, perioral region, and glabella. Nine days later her wounds are reepithelialized and erythema is apparent. Six months later the improvement in facial appearance is evident despite mild hypopigmentation in the perioral region.

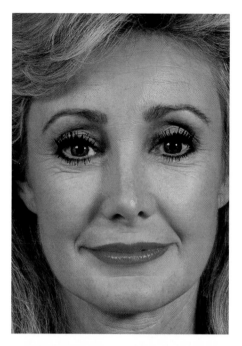

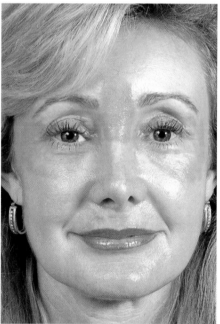
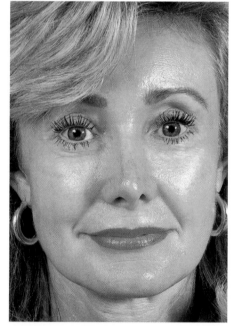

Scanner settings: CPG scanner at 300 mJ with density of 6 × 2 passes for glabella; density of 5 × 2 passes for lower eyelids

This 44-year-old woman exhibits early signs of aging confined to the periorbital area. She had an upper blepharoplasty in conjunction with laser resurfacing of the lower lids, crow's-feet, and glabella. Eight days after treatment reepithelialization and associated erythema can be observed. Three months after treatment healing has progressed, although slight residual erythema requires continued camouflaging makeup and sun avoidance.

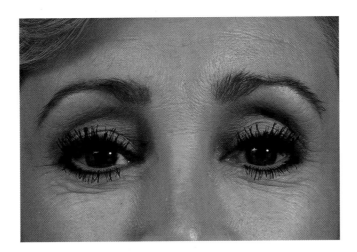

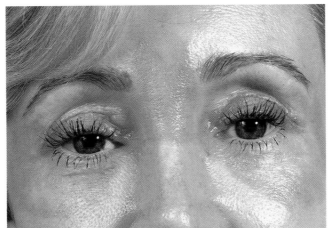

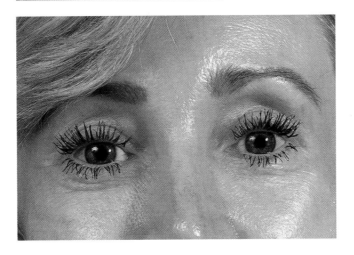

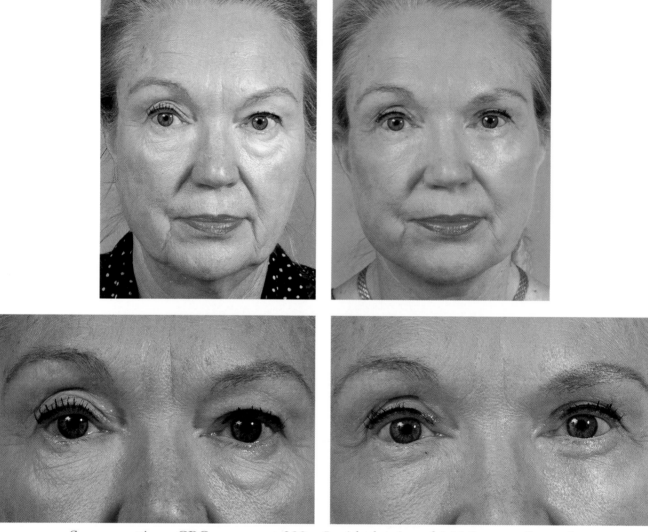

Scanner settings: CPG scanner at 300 mJ with density of 6 × 2 passes for perioral region; density of 5 × 2 passes for lower eyelids

Photoaging and facial laxity are prominent in this patient. The improved results are shown 7 months after she had a face lift, upper blepharoplasty, transconjunctival lower blepharoplasty, and laser resurfacing of the lower lids, crow's-feet, and perioral regions.

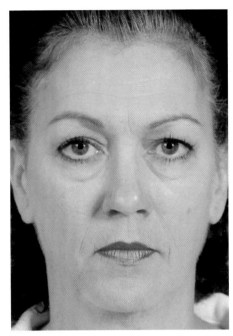 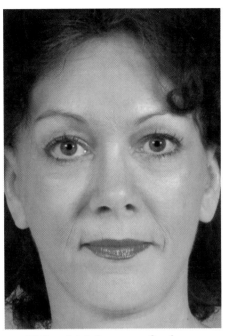

Laser settings: 3 mm Truespot handpiece at 500 mJ × 2 passes for lower eyelids

Patients with herniated lower lid fat, minimal lower lid skin excess, and good lid tone are ideal candidates for transconjunctival blepharoplasty and laser resurfacing. This patient had a face lift, coronal brow lift, transconjunctival blepharoplasty, and laser resurfacing of the lower eyelids. She is seen 2 months after treatment. Note the erythema of the lower lids can be adequately camouflaged with makeup.

COMPLICATIONS AND UNDESIRABLE RESULTS

Hyperpigmentation

The most common complication following laser resurfacing is postinflammatory hyperpigmentation. Virtually all patients will have this problem if they do not use Retin-A and hydroquinone postoperatively and are exposed to sunlight while erythematous. This complication is preventable if proper pretreatment and posttreatment regimens are followed and exposure to sunlight avoided. In the occasional patient who develops postinflammatory hyperpigmentation the addition of kojic acid to the skin care regimen is helpful. Frequent superficial TCA peels are useful adjuncts in treating hyperpigmentation when it is unresponsive to skin creams. Postinflammatory hyperpigmentation will fade in 2 to 6 months in most patients.

Hypopigmentation

A line of demarcation between treated and untreated skin is occasionally noted in patients undergoing regional resurfacing. This probably is the result of the skin returning to its natural color and simply reflects the patient's normal complexion in comparison to adjacent photodamaged skin. Clinically significant hypopigmentation is less common and is most likely related to the depth of injury. When hypopigmentation develops, it is usually most apparent in the perioral region following deep resurfacing and tends to become more noticeable with the passage of time.

Herpes Infection

Similar to other forms of deep resurfacing, herpes infection can occur subsequent to laser resurfacing. Pretreatment with acyclovir or valacyclovir will prevent herpes infection in most patients. If a severe herpes infection should occur, hospitalization and intravenous acyclovir must be considered.

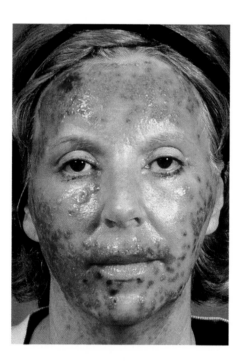

This patient is shown 7 days after full-face laser resurfacing. She was not given prophylactic treatment for herpes infection. She exhibits the classic stigmata of disseminated herpes with vesicle formation, crusting, and pain in the involved areas. She was hospitalized, and intravenous acyclovir, antibiotics, and frequent open wound care initiated. She healed uneventfully. If treated promptly and aggressively, disseminated herpes infections will usually resolve uneventfully.

Scarring

Fortunately hypertrophic scarring has been rare in our experience with laser resurfacing. Proper patient evaluation, adhering to the visual end points in resurfacing, and avoiding resurfacing surgically undermined skin will help prevent this complication. If scarring begins to develop, it must be aggressively treated with low-dose intralesional steroid injections beginning 3 to 4 weeks after treatment. Frequent patient follow-up is necessary to ascertain whether repeated injections are necessary or if silicone sheeting and topical steroids are appropriate.

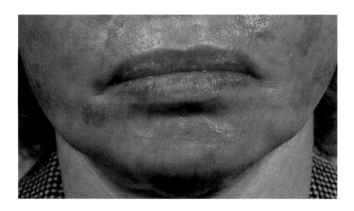

We are seeing a number of patients who have developed hypertropic scarring following laser resurfacing at other clinics. The etiology of scarring is multifactorial. Obviously deep dermal penetration is the primary cause of scarring. Experience is necessary to properly read laser depth in the many varieties of facial skin. When we first started performing laser resurfacing, we took a conservative approach knowing that it was simpler to treat residual rhytides than scarring. Only after performing several hundred laser treatments did we begin to appreciate which skin types could be treated aggressively and those in which conservatism was warranted. We urge physicians just starting to perform laser resurfacing to be cautious. There is a steep learning curve and patience is advised. We recommend beginners use lower energies and fewer passes (even if some wrinkles remain after the procedure is terminated). As experience is gained and the physician becomes comfortable with judging the depth of penetration, more aggressive resurfacing can be attempted.

Lid Retraction and Ectropion

Laser resurfacing of the lower eyelid, especially in elderly patients with poor lid tone, may accentuate lower lid retraction or even produce a frank ectropion. The lower eyelid should be assessed prior to surgery, and if lid tone is poor, a lateral canthoplasty should be performed in conjunction with laser resurfacing.

Many patients will exhibit scleral show immediately following treatment, although this typically resolves in a few weeks as wound healing progresses. Eyelid massage and occasionally taping of the lower eyelid are helpful if lid retraction is severe.

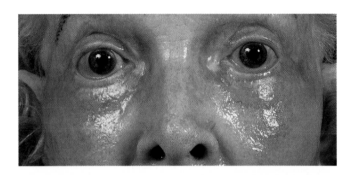

This 80-year-old woman underwent regional resurfacing of the lower eyelid. She is shown 6 weeks following treatment. The significant lower lid retraction and scleral show responded to massage and taping, although it took several months to resolve. A lateral canthoplasty performed in conjunction with resurfacing most likely would have prevented this complication.

Infection

Both bacterial and fungal infections can occur in any open partial-thickness wound. We believe closed dressings are more prone to surface infection and thus we prefer open wound care and frequent wound cleansing. Should infection develop, appropriate cultures must be taken and aggressive parenteral therapy instituted.

Tooth Enamel and Globe Injury

Both the teeth and the eyes must be protected against any possible laser injury. We always use corneal protectors when resurfacing the periorbital region and similarly protect the teeth when resurfacing the mouth.

Prolonged Erythema

All patients will have erythema following laser resurfacing. Erythema typically resolves in 2 to 3 months, although in some individuals it may persist for up to 6 months. Erythema is related to the depth of penetration and is a sign of continued collagen remodeling, new collagen formation, and angiogenesis. If patients do not experience posttreatment erythema, most likely the depth of penetration in resurfacing was limited as will be the long-term result. Deep dermal pathologic conditions require resurfacing into the reticular dermis and thus significant erythema will occur following healing. Although we have never seen a case of permanent erythema, patients can be disturbed by the redness. Reassurance, tincture of time, and occasionally the use of weak steroids (1% hydrocortisone cream) are helpful in patient management. We prefer not to use fluorinated steroids (Temovate) in most patients as it tends to thin the skin and is associated with the development of dermal telangiectasia.

CONCLUDING THOUGHTS

Laser resurfacing represents the newest and most significant tool for facial resurfacing developed in the past 30 years. As with any new technology, experience is required to obtain consistent results. Although the long-term effects of laser resurfacing have yet to be determined, the physician should always remember that the most enduring result in aesthetic surgery is a bad result. In regard to facial resurfacing, hypertropic scars are the most enduring and dreaded sequelae. Secondary procedures are generally successful and usually can be performed at a lighter depth than the original treatment. This should be kept in mind before deciding to perform the last extra pass to treat a recalcitrant facial wrinkle.

Media acceptance of laser resurfacing has brought a host of new patients seeking treatment for photoaged skin. This public demand has stimulated substantial interest, and now many physicians are using lasers to treat actinically damaged skin. This technology has made it possible to improve the appearance of patients who were not candidates for resurfacing in the past. In our enthusiasm to embrace this new technology, however, a word of caution is in order. Let us remember that conservatism and safety must temper our surgical judgment if we are to minimize the potential risk to our patients.

REFERENCES

Alster TS, Apfelberg DB. Cosmetic Laser Surgery. New York: John Wiley & Sons, 1996.

Alster TS, Garg S. Treatment of facial rhytides with a high-energy pulsed carbon dioxide laser. Plast Reconstr Surg 98:791, 1996.

Chernoff G, Schoenrock L, Cramer H, et al. Cutaneous laser resurfacing. Int J Aesthetic Restorative Surg 3:57, 1995.

Cotton J, Hood AF, Gonin R, Deeson WH, Hanke CW. Histologic evaluation of preauricular and postauricular human skin after high-energy short pulsed carbon dioxide laser. Arch Dermatol 132:425, 1996.

David LM. Laser vermilion ablation for actinic cheilitis. J Dermatol Surg Oncol 11:605, 1985.

David LM, Lask GP, Glassberg E, et al. Laser abrasion for cosmetic and medical treatment of facial actinic damage. Cutis 43:583, 1989.

Fitzpatrick RE, Goldman MP. Advances in carbon dioxide laser surgery. Clin Dermatol 13:35, 1995.

Fitzpatrick RE, Ruiz-Esparza JN, Goldman MP. The depth of thermal necrosis using the CO_2 laser: A comparison of the superpulsed mode and conventional modes. J Dermatol Surg Oncol 17: 340, 1991.

Fitzpatrick RE, Goldman MP, Satur N, et al. Pulsed carbon dioxide laser resurfacing of photoaged skin. Arch Dermatol 132:395, 1996.

Goldman MP, Fitzpatrick RE. Cutaneous Laser Surgery. St. Louis: Mosby–Year Book, 1994.

Hobbs E, Bailin P, Wheeland R, Ratz J. Superpulsed lasers: Minimizing thermal damage with short
    duration, high irradiance pulses. J Dermatol Surg Oncol 13:955, 1987.

Hruza GJ. Skin resurfacing with lasers. J Clin Dermatol 3:38, 1995.

Hruza GJ. Laser skin resurfacing. Arch Dermatol 132:451, 1996.

Kamat BR, Tang SU, Arndt KA, et al. Low fluence CO_2 laser irradiation: Selective epidermal dam-
    age to human skin. J Invest Dermatol 85:247, 1995.

Lowe NJ, Lask G, Griffin ME, et al. Skin resurfacing with the UltraPulse carbon dioxide laser.
    Dermatol Surg 21:1025, 1995.

McKenzie AL. How far does thermal damage extend beneath the surface of CO_2 laser incisions?
    Phys Med Biol 28:905, 1983.

Ratz J, McGillis S. Treatment of facial acne scarring with carbon dioxide laser. Am J Cosmet Surg
    9:181, 1992.

Schoenrock LD, Chernoff WG, Rubach BW. Cutaneous UltraPulse laser resurfacing of the eyelids.
    Int J Aesthetic Restorative Surg 3:31, 1995.

Seckel BR. Aesthetic Laser Surgery. Boston: Little, Brown, 1996.

Stuzin JM, Baker TJ, Baker TM, Kligman AM. Histologic effects of the high-energy pulsed CO_2
    laser on photoaged facial skin. Plast Reconstr Surg 99:2036, 1997.

Walsh JT, Flotte TJ, Anderson RR, et al. Pulsed CO_2 laser tissue ablation: Effect of tissue type and
    pulse duration on thermal damage. Lasers Surg Med 8:108, 1989.

Weinstein C. UltraPulse carbon dioxide laser removal of periocular wrinkles in association with laser
    blepharoplasty. J Clin Laser Med Surg 12:205, 1994.

Yang CC, Chai CY. Animal study of skin resurfacing using the UltraPulse carbon dioxide laser. Ann
    Plast Surg 35:154, 1995.

Index